THE FITNESS BOOK
For People With Diabetes

A project of
The American Diabetes Association Council On Exercise

W. Guyton Hornsby, Jr., PhD, CDE, *Editor in Chief*
West Virginia University

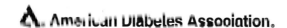
American Diabetes Association.

Publisher
Susan H. Lau

Editorial Director
Peter Banks

Managing Editor
Christine B. Welch

Associate Editor
Sherrye Landrum

Printed in the United States of America

AMERICAN DIABETES ASSOCIATION
1660 Duke Street
Alexandria, Virginia 22314

Library of Congress Cataloging-in-Publication Data

The Fitness book for people with diabetes
W. Guyton Hornsby, Jr., editor in chief
p. cm.
Includes index.

1. Diabetes—Exercise therapy. 2. Physical fitness. I. Hornsby,
W. Guyton. II. American Diabetes Association.
RC661.E94F56 1994
616.4'62062—dc20   93-43785

ISBN 0-945448-33-3 (pbk.)

TABLE OF CONTENTS

FOREWORD by Chris Silkwood vi
ACKNOWLEDGMENTS viii
CONTRIBUTORS...ix

CHAPTER 1: THE VALUE OF EXERCISE 1
   Why Aren't You Exercising? 2
   Background on Diabetes..2
   Why All People With Diabetes Need to Exercise 2
   Diabetes Complications and Exercise...5
   If Diabetes Runs in Your Family, Read This..6
   Ready, Set, Go! 6

CHAPTER 2: GETTING YOUR MIND READY TO EXERCISE............................7
   Self-Motivation Is Best...8
   Assessing Your Program 8
   Sticking With It 14

CHAPTER 3: GETTING YOUR BODY READY TO EXERCISE 17
   Your Preexercise Physical 18
   Exercise Testing...22

CHAPTER 4: YOUR EXERCISE PRESCRIPTION 31
   What Should I Do? 33
   How Hard Should I Exercise? 35
   How Long Should I Exercise? 41
   How Often Should I Exercise? 41
   Where Do I Start? 43
   Keeping an Exercise Log 43

CHAPTER 5: EXERCISING SAFELY 47

Exercise and Blood Glucose Levels..48
Going Low 48
Going High 49
You Don't Self-Monitor? Read This...52
How Blood Glucose Levels Respond to Exercise 57
Tailoring Your Glucose Control Plan 57
Insulin Action During Exercise 58
Listening to Your Body 59
Diet-Managed Diabetes and Blood Glucose 60
Avoiding Exercise Injury..61
Drink Plenty of Fluids...61
Keeping One Foot Ahead of Problems 62
Dress for the Weather 64

CHAPTER 6: EXERCISING TO INCREASE YOUR FITNESS 65

Getting Aerobically Fit..66
Strength Training 72
Activities to Improve Flexibility 76
Training With Machines 83
Where Should I Exercise?..89

CHAPTER 7: EXERCISING TO LOSE WEIGHT.......................................91

How Exercise Helps You Lose Weight..92
The Link Between Diabetes and Body Weight 92
Exercise for Beginners...93
Aerobics and Weight Loss...97
But Exercise Makes Me Hungry!..97
The Myths About Dieting...97
Making Changes in Your Diet 99
Staying Motivated 103

CHAPTER 8: EXERCISING WITH SPECIAL NEEDS 105
   Exercise for the Older Generations...106
   Diabetes Complications 111
   Exercise After Transplantation..119
   Exercise and Pregnancy...122

CHAPTER 9: COMPETING WITH DIABETES 125
   Do You Have What It Takes? 126
   Team Sports 126
   How Do You See Your Diabetes?..127
   The Keys to Athletic Success 130
   Fueling Up 131
   Carbohydrate Replacement 133
   High-Risk Sports—A Personal Choice 136

GLOSSARY 139
RESOURCES 140
INDEX 146

FOREWORD

ONE OF THE MOST DIFFICULT CHALLENGES IN LIFE IS TO ACCEPT THE THINGS YOU CANNOT CONTROL. No one wants to have diabetes. In fact, most of us would love to snap our fingers and have it instantly go away. The good news, however, is that diabetes can be managed and complications minimized if you are willing to practice a healthy lifestyle.

I have chosen to accept diabetes as an opportunity. I know that, because of my diabetes and my commitment to good health through regular exercise and a healthy diet, I am in better shape than most of my friends who take their health for granted.

Because of diabetes, you run a higher than normal risk of developing disease in the most important muscle in your body: your heart. Exercise is a fun way to improve the health of your heart and maintain its function as a strong pump. Increased heart rates during exercise activity will boost oxygen use and help burn up calories.

Exercise has numerous benefits: it can help you control blood glucose levels, improve your health, and make you feel better about yourself. Regular aerobic activity, such as brisk walking, cycling, or swimming, reduces excess body fat, strengthens the heart and blood vessels, lowers cholesterol and blood glucose, and serves as a constructive outlet for stress.

Stress is a factor in everyone's life. How you channel stress influences how it affects your body. Typically, high stress levels will raise blood glucose levels. There's nothing like a brisk walk or a bicycle ride to relieve stress and calm your nerves.

Feeling good is an essential part of staying healthy. Even on those tough days when you'd rather be doing anything else but exercising, try to push yourself a bit and do it anyway. Motivation is the key. If you choose an exercise program that you enjoy, and develop some skill at it, chances are you will keep doing it. Take the time to enjoy a "shopping spree" with exercise. Try many types of activities in a variety of environments. You may find that an enthusiastic exercise leader makes an aerobics class fun, or that a jog or walk in the park is more suitable for you. Or you may prefer teaming up with a personal trainer.

Listen to your own body and don't overexercise. The old notion of having to "go for the burn" just isn't true. You should be pleasantly tired after an exercise routine, not totally fatigued. Always exercise at the level of your ability and don't compete with your classmates or your instructor.

Regular exercise has helped me fulfill many of my diabetes management goals. Most important, exercise has given me the sense of "being in control." I am more in tune with my body and more aware of its needs and its physiological changes. As a result, I'm far more demanding in the cause of my own good health.

Make exercise a part of your daily routine. I've made a routine of testing my blood glucose before exercise and snacking as needed. I never exercise without some form of "quick sugar" in my pocket, regardless of my starting blood glucose level. I try to exercise at about the same time each day. I exercise each evening after work and on weekends before dinner, which means I work out seven days a week. Even if exercising every day is unrealistic for you, try not to let more than two days pass without working out. Although I exercise every day, I don't always work out at full intensity; some days I play tennis or another recreational sport just for fun.

Exercise is a gift you can give to yourself. Reserve some time each day to take care of yourself by exercising. You are worth it! And exercise is an absolute must for quality diabetes management. Do yourself a great favor and begin an exercise program today.

Chris Silkwood, BS, Exercise Physiology
Director, Diabetes Treatment Centers of America/Park Plaza Hospital
Member, President's Council on Physical Fitness and Sports

ACKNOWLEDGMENTS

This book was truly a group effort. In 1990, the American Diabetes Association Council on Exercise pointed out the need to help people with diabetes exercise safely and effectively. Oversight of the project was given to council member Guyton Hornsby, Jr., PhD, CDE, an exercise physiologist who works in a university setting. It is due to Guy's efforts that this book can claim to be the best source of information available to people with diabetes about exercise. He asked other council members who had volunteered to work on the project to write about topics such as motivation, safety, exercise testing, and exercising with complications. The ten contributors (see list) did not let their interest and enthusiasm for the project waver even as they were asked to rewrite, review, and wait patiently to see the results of their labor.

Managing editor Christine Welch rewrote and shaped these topics into chapters that would invite the reader to know the joy and benefits of exercise and to create an individually tailored exercise program. During this process, writers Craig Steinburg and Amanda Patton contributed talent and effort. Amanda interviewed those people with diabetes whom you meet in the pages of this book. Associate editor Sherrye Landrum kept track of photographs, resources, and numerous drafts as the editing and production process unfolded.

We thank the reviewers who shared their comments with us: Ann Cabanas, RD, LD, MPH, University of Texas Medical Branch; Barbara N. Campaigne, PhD, FACSM, American College of Sports Medicine; Mark Feinglos, MD, Duke University Medical Center; Neal Friedman, MD, Lovelace Medical Center; David B. Kelley, MD; and Paula Yutzy, RN, CDE.

Each of the following people in some way helped finish *The Fitness Book*. Thanks go to Carol Segree, Richard Kahn, PhD, Peter Banks, Phyllis Barrier, RD, CDE, Steve Prosterman, Christine Silkwood, Anne Riley, RN, CDE, Dorothy Efland, Carol Gibson, Patricia Painter, PhD, F. Xavier, Pi-Sunyer, MD, Gerald Rogell, MD, and Janet Wallace, PhD. We are also grateful to the people we profiled, who graciously agreed to tell you about their relationship with exercise and diabetes.

Illustrations were drawn by Elizabeth Ann Jordan. Page design and desktop publishing services were provided by Insight Graphics, Inc. Cover design is by Wickham & Associates, Inc.

CONTRIBUTORS

EDITOR IN CHIEF
W. Guyton Hornsby, Jr., PhD, CDE
West Virginia University
Morgantown, West Virginia

CONTRIBUTING EDITORS

William Coleman, DPM
Oschner Clinic
New Orleans, Louisiana

John T. Devlin, MD
Maine Medical Center
Portland, Maine

Marion Franz, MS, RD, CDE
International Diabetes Center
Minneapolis, Minnesota

Claudia Graham, PhD, MPH, CDE
Diabetes Management Center at
Presbyterian Intercommunity Hospital
Whittier, California

Yolanda Groenewoud, MD, FRCPC
Mount Sinai Hospital
Toronto, Ontario, Canada

Paula Harper, RN, CDE
International Diabetic Athletes
Association
Phoenix, Arizona

David Marrero, PhD
Regenstrief Institute
Indianapolis, Indianapolis

Stephen Schneider, MD, FACP
R. Wood Johnson Medical School
New Brunswick, New Jersey

Irma Ullrich, MD
West Virginia University
Morgantown, West Virginia

Bernard Zinman, MD, FACP
Mount Sinai Hospital
Toronto, Ontario, Canada

Fitness means you are ready to do anything. To be fit is to be sound physically and mentally, to be healthy, and adaptable to every new condition that comes into your life.

The *Value* of Exercise

HOW MANY THINGS DO WE DO DAY AFTER DAY, EVERY DAY? We wake up, dress ourselves, eat, and wash. We drive, work, talk, think, laugh, plan ahead. We sleep. And those of us with diabetes treat ourselves every day.

Diabetes is a daily disease. It is a life-long disease. We look at diabetes as an added dimension to our days, which is sometimes a challenge and at other times a burden. The daily responsibility for our diabetes care belongs to us.

Those of us who have made the decision to live a long and healthy life despite diabetes have something in common. We exercise.

WHY AREN'T YOU EXERCISING?

Exercise makes you feel good and look great. Regular exercise is important for everyone's good health.

- It gives you more energy.
- It strengthens your heart.
- It improves your circulation.
- It strengthens your muscles.
- It increases your flexibility.
- It improves your breathing.
- It helps you manage your weight.
- It delays the effects of aging.
- It improves blood pressure.
- It improves cholesterol and other blood fats.
- It lessens stress.
- It counteracts the effects of inactivity.

On top of all this, exercise is fun! When you increase your fitness, you improve your health and appearance. You will feel better about yourself. So do something good for yourself! Get up and get moving!

Hold on! Because exercise affects the very thing you need to control—your blood glucose level—you have a lot of questions about exercise. It's important for you to exercise safely. You also need to know how to reach your particular fitness goals, such as losing weight, improving your overall health, or competing in a community health run or walk, while managing your diabetes.

BACKGROUND ON DIABETES

Exercise and fitness are key ingredients in diabetes self-care. This is because your level of fitness affects the body's metabolism—how it captures and uses energy. Diabetes is a metabolic disease.

Diabetes changes the way your body gets energy from foods. The problem in diabetes is that the body loses its ability to store carbohydrates, proteins, and fats. This is because insulin is missing or ineffective. Insulin is a "storage" hormone—it allows fuels, primarily glucose from food, to enter the body's cells to be used or stored. The key feature of diabetes is a blood glucose level that is higher than normal. This is a sign that insulin is not doing its job.

In insulin-dependent (type I) diabetes, the pancreas stops making insulin. People with type I diabetes must get their insulin from insulin injections. If no insulin, or not enough insulin, is available in the body, two problems result: 1) the level of glucose in the blood is high, a condition called hyperglycemia, and 2) the body is forced to break down excess amounts of stored fat for energy. Both of these problems are unhealthy for the body.

In non-insulin-dependent (type II) diabetes, the pancreas makes insulin, but it is not released or used properly by the body. The cells don't respond as they should to insulin, a condition called insulin resistance. This leads to high blood glucose levels. Sometimes, oral medications or insulin injections are needed by people with type II diabetes to overcome insulin resistance. In many people, insulin resistance appears to be worsened by being overweight. Losing weight with diet and exercise reduces insulin resistance and lowers blood glucose levels.

WHY ALL PEOPLE WITH DIABETES NEED TO EXERCISE

Exercise is beneficial to the health of people with both types of diabetes in two ways: 1) it can take some glucose out of the blood to use for energy during and after exercise, which lowers blood glucose levels, and 2) it helps delay or stop large blood vessel and heart (cardiovascular) disease. Cardiovascular disease is the leading killer of people with diabetes. All people with diabetes should exercise to counteract their increased risk for cardiovascular disease, to reach and stay at a healthy weight, and to enjoy themselves. These are the main reasons why exercise is so important for people with diabetes. Exercise has an additional benefit for many people with diabetes: exercise (plus other healthy lifestyle habits) can help them achieve good blood glucose control. When blood glucose levels are as near to normal as possible, small blood vessel disease, which affects the eyes and kidneys, and nerve damage due to diabetes can be delayed or halted.

If you have type II diabetes, regular exercise is one of the best ways to manage your disease. Exercise should be prescribed in your treatment plan, along with a healthy meal plan and medications, if needed. It can help you overcome the basic problem that causes your blood glucose level to be too high. As you increase your energy output with exercise, not only do you increase the fitness of your heart, lungs, and muscles, but you also train your body to use insulin more efficiently. Increasing your insulin "fitness" improves your blood glucose control. Exercise is a tool you can use to help control your blood glucose level. Regular exercise is also recommended for treatment of type II diabetes because it reduces your risk of cardiovascular disease, can help you feel better, and can help you control your weight.

Where does fitness fit into type I diabetes care? Exercise is very important for people with type I diabetes because it reduces the risk of cardiovascular disease by improving overall fitness and improves the body's response to insulin. Exercising to increase or maintain your fitness will not change your need to carefully balance insulin with food and exercise. If you do not adjust your plan to account for exercise, such as eating enough extra food to match the calories you use during your workout, you could develop dangerously low blood glucose levels. Exercise can also lead to hyperglycemia and possibly ketosis (a build-up of acids in body tissues and fluids) if you don't have enough insulin available. You should receive an exercise prescription to aid you in learning how exercise affects your blood glucose levels and your insulin and meal plans.

To manage type I diabetes, you must supply your body with insulin as it needs it. The pancreas has a job that is lost in type I diabetes that you may not think about: it pays attention to the glucose levels in your body, minute to minute, and releases insulin as needed. Unfortunately, there is no good way for you to perform this job as well as a healthy pancreas can. Your best substitute is to monitor your blood glucose levels and have an individualized diabetes care plan that matches your food and activity.

Whether you have type I or type II diabetes, there are very good reasons why you should take the extra effort to include exercise in your diabetes management. Reducing your risk of cardiovascular disease and increasing your body's efficient use of insulin (you may need less insulin because of exercise) may be reasons you care about. Taking insulin injections shouldn't keep you in an easy chair or on the sidelines. You should allow yourself to do any activity that is reasonable for you—anything from daily walks with your family or friends to competitive sports with the team. Along the way, you will notice other benefits, like improvements

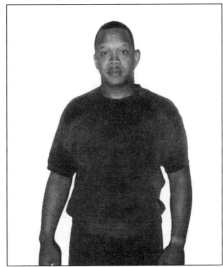

"**Y**OU HAVE TO BUILD UP SLOWLY." Ask Ron Ball about fitness, and he'll tell you he's been involved "practically all my life." He grew up loving Little League baseball and football. At 13, he became interested in karate. Fourteen years in the U.S. Marine Corps bolstered his commitment to staying fit.

Ron still makes fitness a priority. His daily workouts include stretching, some cardiovascular warm up, and weight training. He works out several times a week at a karate school near his home.

But recently, Ron has had to grapple with a new challenge to staying fit—being diagnosed with diabetes. The diagnosis was not a total surprise; both of Ron's parents had diabetes. He also had a frightening warning—he suffered a mild stroke two weeks before being diagnosed.

"I was feeling bad and thought I was dehydrated," he says. "I thought maybe if I drank a lot of water I'd feel better." When they checked his blood glucose level at the hospital, it was more than 800 mg/dl. Ron spent four days in the hospital, learning about diabetes. "I took classes on nutrition...and classes on diabetes management." He learned about checking blood glucose levels with a meter. Ron is able to control his diabetes with oral medication.

While at the VA hospital, Ron talked to his doctors about exercise. He says they were supportive of his continuing to work out. They suggested he start back slowly and talked to him about the importance of taking good care of his feet.

Ron gradually rebuilt his exercise program. "When something like diabetes happens to you, it takes a lot out of you. You have to build up again slowly." Today, he enjoys working out at the karate club because "subconsciously when you work out by yourself you have a tendency to cheat. You don't do full reps [repetitions], full sets. People there will help you out. Count for you."

In addition to his full-time job, Ron occasionally moonlights as a bodyguard for entertainers performing in the Washington, D.C., area. He's guarded such rap artists as LL Cool, Johnny Gill, and Crystal Water. Regular workouts keep him in top shape for these high-pressure assignments.

After several years with diabetes, Ron is still learning how to plan for low blood glucose reactions after exercise. He's found that drinking Gatorade during his workouts helps. He also keeps candy nearby.

Ron admits that adjusting to having diabetes can be a psychological hurdle. He believes that "it's just a matter of trying to get used to it. Sometimes you feel you can't do what other people can do, but you can. You can." ∎

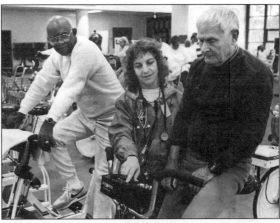

Stationary bikes are one tool for increasing fitness.
Photograph by Les Todd, Courtesy of Duke University Photo Department.

in your appearance and in your self-esteem. You'll also have a fun way to unwind and enjoy being with other people.

DIABETES COMPLICATIONS AND EXERCISE

Most everyone with diabetes has been introduced to the term *diabetes complications*. These are health problems that develop over time because of diabetes. Some complications are a direct result of living with abnormally high blood glucose levels. There can be damage to fine capillary beds and small blood vessels in the kidneys and eyes as well as to the nervous system.

High blood glucose levels in combination with abnormal insulin levels, high blood pressure, and an imbalance of blood fats can also affect the large blood vessels. Diabetes often leads to heart disease, circulation problems, and strokes. To combat large blood vessel disease, exercise has been shown to reduce cardiovascular disease risk by lowering blood pressure and blood lipid levels.

Small blood vessel disease can be delayed or slowed dramatically with tight blood glucose control. This was proven in the Diabetes Control and Complications Trial (DCCT), a 10-year study of people with type I diabetes. It showed that the closer to normal your blood glucose level is, the lower your risk of disease of the eyes, kidneys, and nerves. Achieving normal blood glucose levels is not easy and requires very intensive diabetes treatment. The "intensively" managed subjects in the DCCT gained an average of 10 pounds more and had significantly more serious low blood glucose (hypoglycemic) reactions than subjects managed with standard care. Although tight control is not the best treatment for everyone, it does appear that most people should attempt to get blood glucose levels as close to normal as possible.

Exercise alone will not improve glucose control in type I diabetes. Increased exercise should help keep your weight under control with intensive management, but hypoglycemia is a very real risk. Adding exercise to your diabetes care plan will require the careful balance of food, insulin, and physical activity. You and your health-care team—your physician, a nurse educator, a dietitian, and perhaps other specialists such as an exercise physiologist, a podiatrist, and an ophthalmologist—should work together to find out what's best for you. There are strategies to get good blood glucose control and still let you lead an active life that promotes fitness.

Although people with type II diabetes were not studied in the DCCT, the risk reduction for small blood vessel and nerve disease that comes with good blood glucose control may apply to people with type II diabetes, too. People with type II diabetes can help control their blood glucose level with exercise.

Exercise can make many improvements in your health that help balance out your risk for diabetes complications. For instance, a program of regular exercise lowers blood pressure. Because high blood pressure also damages capillary beds in the eyes and kidneys, keeping blood pressure normal can keep your eyes and kidneys in better shape. Controlling blood pressure is also important in preventing heart disease and strokes.

Exercise lowers high levels of triglycerides and low-density lipoprotein (LDL) cholesterol, blood fats that can clog arteries and damage the heart. Over time, regular exercise increases the level of high density lipoprotein (HDL) cholesterol, which helps protect against large blood vessel disease. Exercise helps improve blood flow throughout the body. Improving blood flow in the feet and legs is especially important in diabetes.

IF DIABETES RUNS IN YOUR FAMILY, READ THIS

Do you have a grandparent, parent, sister, or brother with type II diabetes? If so, chances are greater than usual that you and other members of your family will develop type II diabetes. The tendency to inherit this disease is high.

Does this mean that you're destined to develop diabetes if it runs in your family? No! Exercise can help protect you from ever developing type II diabetes. Regular exercise fights insulin resistance and obesity, allowing people to avoid developing diabetes in the first place.

Researchers believe that this is due to the effect exercise can have on insulin sensitivity. Type II diabetes may come on slowly, over a period of several years. During this time, the body requires more and more insulin to overcome insulin resistance. But having high levels of insulin in the body makes the body less sensitive to insulin. When you participate in regular exercise, your body becomes more sensitive to the insulin that's available. Eventually, you won't need as much insulin as you used to…and the type II diabetes can be prevented or made easier to manage.

In addition, even if your family members never develop type II diabetes, they are at increased risk of the accompanying health problems such as high blood pressure and blood lipid levels. Exercise can bring this risk down.

If you have type II diabetes, encourage your relatives, especially your children, to exercise with you. If you develop an active lifestyle, your family probably will, too. It's the best present you could possibly give them.

READY, SET, GO!

Your first steps toward a more active lifestyle should begin with a thorough medical examination. This is the only way to make sure your exercise program meets your individual needs.

One exercise program does not fit all! Everyone is different, and your exercise plan has to be based on your health and your body's needs. For example, you may have a back problem, high blood pressure, bad knees, or weak ankles. Or you may already have some diabetes complications—a faster than normal heart beat, clogged blood vessels in the heart, eye disease, or nerve damage. Working with your health-care team will give you the confidence of knowing that you're doing all you can to avoid the pitfalls and reap only the benefits of exercise.

A healthy, active lifestyle is a lifetime plan. For an exercise program to be beneficial, you must faithfully stick to it. Pounds lost will return and lowered blood pressure will become high again if you stop exercising. So choose activities that you enjoy, that are convenient to do, and that are right for your level of fitness.

There are many ways to stay active. For most of us, a comfortable walk or bike ride is the answer. An exercise plan doesn't have to include marathon running or high-powered aerobics unless that's what you're really suited for and like to do. Being active is supposed to be fun, not a struggle. You just have to find what's right for you.

*It does not matter
so much where we
are as the direction
we are moving.*
—Goethe

CHAPTER 2

Getting Your *Mind* Ready to Exercise

YOU KNOW ALL THE REASONS WHY YOU SHOULD
BEGIN TO EXERCISE, but there's actually only one
reason for making it a habit—because it makes you
feel good. A fit body lives up to its potential. Your
body is your own miracle machine, specially made to
move you through the world, feeling all of the sensations that
life can offer. Well-used muscles stimulate your brain with new
kinds of information. This helps balance other types of mental
exercises, such as money worries or family problems.

If you're used to feeling uncomfortable in your body, you

can change that. You may have been trying to run away from your body ever since you got embarrassed in school gym class, or put on too many pounds, or reached a certain birthday, or got diabetes. But you can't get fit by running away. You get fit by moving your body through the air, through the water, over the floor, or out the door. People give many reasons for why they don't get any exercise. They say they're too tired, or too old, or too fat, or too uncoordinated, or too busy. They may be afraid they'll hurt themselves or look silly. But none of these excuses stands in the way of someone who intends to make a change. Even with an injury or disability, there are ways to improve fitness.

There are as many different ways to improve your fitness as there are personalities. The best activities are the ones you like, because those are the ones you'll do. So, explore and find out what you like. You'll feel awkward, uncomfortable, and perhaps anxious when you try something new, but everyone does. Learn a new way to exercise from someone who loves it and ease yourself into it. Then you'll rediscover the joy of play!

SELF-MOTIVATION IS THE BEST

A good place to start is in your mind. What are your intentions? If you have type II diabetes, you've probably been told that exercise will improve your diabetes control or help you lose weight. These are good reasons, and they may get you started, but they might not be good enough reasons to keep you motivated. Dig a little deeper inside and decide what you could gain from regular exercise. Perhaps you want to improve your appearance. Maybe you like the competition of sports or simply enjoy the camaraderie of teammates. Maybe you like the escape that exercise time gives you away from the day-to-day grind.

You can take a cue from many successful large corporations who develop mission statements that—in a few words—explain the basic philosophy of the business and what they want to achieve. They've found that defining what their companies are about, why they are in business, and what they hope to achieve helps employees to have a sense of purpose and a direction to take. You can develop your own mission statement that will help you define just what you hope to achieve through exercise. For example, your fitness mission statement might be something like: "I strive to live a healthy lifestyle so that I feel good and have the energy to accomplish my daily and lifetime goals." The whole idea is to find and state your reasons for exercising, not someone else's.

The next step is to select activities that will fit your needs and that you find enjoyable. Some exercises may turn out to feel like pure drudgery while others you'll find you really enjoy. The odds are good that you will stick to activities that you enjoy. Some people enjoy their daily walks by window shopping. Others spend time on the exercise bike or other equipment during a favorite television show or while listening to cheerful music on a headset.

ASSESSING YOUR PROGRAM

A good way to determine whether the exercise you choose has a good chance of succeeding is to put it to a test. Think about how you would answer the following questions. They should help you decide what activities are realistic for you and fit your needs and lifestyle.

First, think about convenience.

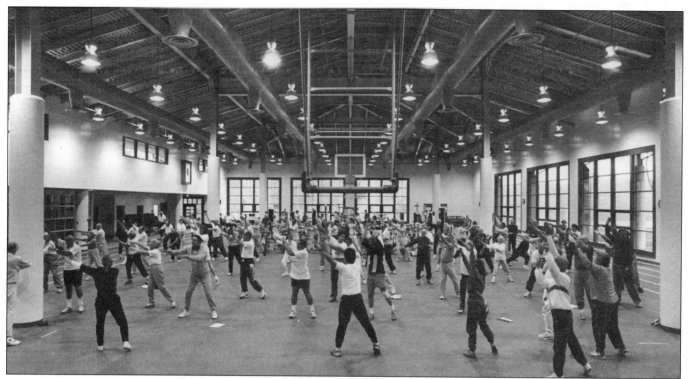

Group workouts can keep you motivated. Photograph by Les Todd, courtesy of Duke University Photo Department.

Do you need special facilities to do it? If you want to swim and don't have a pool, you'll need to find a facility with one. If you want to participate in an aerobics class, you'll need to go where the class is offered. Find out about the facility. Is it near your work or home? Is it easy to get to? Can you afford the monthly or yearly fees? Is it a place in which you feel comfortable?

Does it require special equipment? Many sports or exercises require special equipment. Do you have access to the equipment you need? Will you need to purchase the equipment? Can you afford it? For example, a good pair of running shoes can cost about $60 to $100. A bicycle can cost even more. Do you want to make such an investment? Don't try to make do with equipment that is in bad shape or ill suited to the exercise you are doing. It could be a sure invitation to injury—one of the biggest barriers to motivation. Besides, one of the neatest things about sports is the gear that goes with them.

Does it require special training? Some activities require you to learn correct techniques to ensure that

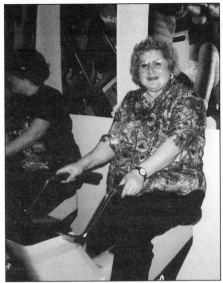

"I'M A SHOW-ME KIND OF PERSON."

For Carol Schwartz, seeing was believing. Part of the diabetes education program that she attended focused on the importance of exercise to manage diabetes. Before walking on a treadmill, the class tested their blood glucose. They tested again after exercising and blood glucose levels were lower. "I guess I'm a show-me kind of person," says Carol. "The work on the treadmill proved to me that there was a definite correlation between exercising and lowering my blood glucose."

When Carol signed up for that education program five years ago, diabetes was not new in her life. She had already had the disease for ten years. However, at the time, her mother, who also had diabetes, was terminally ill with cancer. Stress was beginning to affect Carol's control, and she felt the week-long education program would help her. "Being an RN, I knew pretty much about the diabetic disease process. I knew how to take injections and regulate medications. Exercise was the new part," says Carol.

Finding a way to work exercise into her everyday life proved difficult. Carol started on a walking program but after a while had trouble staying motivated. She'd always enjoyed bowling, but the recreational sport was not vigorous or sustained enough to provide an aerobic workout.

She also had to find a way to squeeze exercise into an already brimming schedule. As a public health nurse, Carol spends most of her days traveling to the homes of elderly patients. In addition to working full-time, she attends college part-time, working toward a degree in health-care administration. Then, she has her family responsibilities as well.

Joining a health club seems to have helped Carol stay focused on regular exercise. "Believe it or not, I think I'm going because I paid for it," says Carol. "Because I'm paying for a particular service, I want to get my money's worth."

Carol comes home from work, eats dinner, and then goes to the gym. She joined the health club with a friend; she found making the commitment with a buddy helpful. Carol tries to make it to the gym three times a week. Typically, she rides a stationary bike and does a routine with weights. She might also work out on a stairclimber machine. She's generally finished in about an hour. Although her primary exercise goal is fitness, she'd also like to shed a few pounds.

For Carol, nothing speaks louder than seeing the results of her exercise efforts. She joined the health club this past spring. "I had started exercising June 14th. At the end of the first week in July, I had an appointment with my doctor. I had to have blood work done. After two weeks of exercising, my cholesterol level had dropped from 220 to 169," says Carol. With benefits like those after only a few weeks, Carol figures months or years of regular exercise will only make things better. ∎

you do them safely. Weight lifting is a good example. If you've never participated in a weight lifting program, have someone who has been certified by the National Strength and Conditioning Association (look for the designation CSCS after their name) or another exercise organization (see Chapter 6) show you how to properly lift the weights. Lifting them wrong could put an unnecessary strain on your body and cause injuries that would slow down your fitness schedule. Cross-country skiing takes some skill and a few lessons will get you off on the right foot. Even your running stride could be improved by learning the right techniques from an expert.

Do you need others to exercise with you? There are a number of terrific sports that require one or more people to play. But will you always be able to find a partner when you want (or need) to play? If you want to exercise regularly, you'll need to find people with the same desire and schedule as yours who will be available and willing when you are. A family member or neighbor might be a good choice.

Is it seasonal? Many activities are, by their nature or by your location, seasonal. Cross-country skiing is one. Swimming is another if you don't have an indoor pool available. Running could be seasonal if the temperatures in your area get dangerously hot or cold. To keep up a regular exercise program, you need to have alternative activities that you enjoy in the off-season.

Now do some thinking about your physical attributes and lifestyle.

Do you have physical limitations? Before you start to exercise, know your limits. How you exercise will depend on your weight and fitness level, any injuries or conditions you have, and whether you have complications from diabetes. For example, maybe you'd like to start a running program but have bad knees. After a few weeks or days of running, your body will tell you it's time to call it quits. Instead, you might consider swimming or pedalling a stationary recumbent bike—exercises that don't put excess stress on your knees. If you have hypertension and want to work out with weights, you need to be shown how to breathe and perform the lifts correctly to avoid problems.

There is nothing more important to your health than your preexercise physical exam. If you haven't exercised in a while, for instance a year, a preexercise exam is a necessity. It's also necessary if you've had any changes in your health status, like development of a diabetes complication or worsening of blood glucose control. If you're used to exercising, but want to begin a new activity, consult with your health-care team.

Can you realistically integrate the activity into your lifestyle? One of the biggest barriers to maintaining a long-term exercise program is finding the time to do it. Many of us will plan to exercise only to find that the competing demands of our lives make it difficult or even impossible. If you have to make too many adjustments to get an exercise routine into your schedule, you probably won't be able to do it. You are more likely to maintain a program that smoothly meshes with your everyday routine. For example, if you normally sleep in to the last possible minute in the morning, making plans to rise an hour earlier every day to work out is unrealistic! Likewise, the varied demands of your family may make establishing a schedule difficult.

In situations where time is difficult to find, remember that you don't have to devote several hours a day to exercise effectively. Twenty to 45 minutes every other day will benefit your overall fitness. If you're out to lose

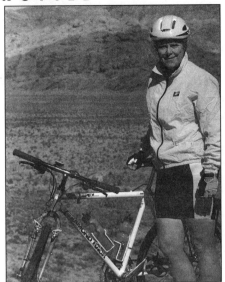

"I JUST DECIDED I'M NOT LETTING ANYTHING GET ME DOWN."

When Delores Nardone was diagnosed with type II diabetes in August 1989, it was not exactly a surprise. She was 52 years old and weighed 265 pounds. Her grandfather had died of diabetes-related complications, and her mother also had the disease. Perhaps because she'd seen the ravages diabetes can inflict firsthand, the diagnosis was difficult to accept. She came home from the doctor's office depressed and feeling sorry for herself. Her doctor had given her an 800-calorie diet and medication and told her to come back in a couple of weeks to check the dosage.

It didn't take long for Delores's natural optimism to assert itself, however. A major morale boost came from a hospital diabetes education program that her husband encouraged her to attend. She credits the program with saving her life. "They gave me the information to understand how to take charge of this disease," she says. "I learned so much. The dietitian immediately called my doctor and asked permission to put me on a 1200-calorie diet. I knew I had to take charge of my diabetes. I'm a very positive person, and I just decided I'm not letting anything get me down."

The diabetes education program met for an hour and a half a day for five days and was offered free of charge. Through the program Delores learned how to monitor her blood glucose, the importance of exercise, and, as she says, "the dirty end of diabetes...what can happen if you're not good. They laid it on the line."

Fired up by the program, Delores began to walk for exercise. She started slowly, working up to one mile and then two miles. She also decided to make weight loss a challenge. "I had been praying for a diet I could live with, and no matter how hard I tried I couldn't do it. Then I learned that I had diabetes and if I wanted to live, I'd better diet. I decided that if I had to diet I'd see how long it would take me to lose 100 pounds by diet and exercise. I was on 1200 calo-

ries a day, and I did not cheat. My exercise was no more than walking two miles around the block and later biking two miles. It doesn't take a lot of exercise to control your blood glucose."

Delores even made testing her blood glucose into a game. She found that she had to cut back on her medication because exercise was lowering her blood glucose. "In the beginning I was testing a bunch. It was so exciting to watch my body come into control." Eventually, she was able to go off medication entirely.

When Delores got down to 200 pounds, she started biking. "It was comical," she says. "My son brought his mountain bike over and my husband said, `I want you to try this.' I said, 'No way.'" Not only did Delores wind up riding her son's bike, her husband Tom decided to keep her company on her workouts. "He didn't want me out there on the street by myself, so he started going out with me." Eating healthier meals along with Delores, Tom lost about 40 pounds. "Now he's more of a fanatic than I am," laughs Delores.

With her weight down to 165 pounds, Delores put herself to the challenge of a 150-mile bike-a-thon. The event, which raised funds for charity, featured a bike route stretching from Las Vegas to the London Bridge in Lake Havasu, Nevada. Competitors would have to ride 95 miles the first day and 55 the next. Delores conned herself into entering by telling herself that she wouldn't have to finish. But, in fact, once she registered and collected pledges, she felt a growing commitment to the ride. She trained carefully, gradually increasing her mileage. Not only did she finish the two-day event, but she wrote an essay about her struggle with diabetes. That essay won her the 1990 Catfish Hunter Hall of Fame Award.

But there's more to Delores's story. Like most people with type II diabetes, she is still fighting a constant battle with the scales. She's gained back some weight but remains optimistic and energetic in her battle for control. "It's tough to stay motivated," she says. "That's why I've let my weight go back up." Currently at 215 pounds, she says she's been "rocking back and forth for about six months." Still, she says, "I have to get up in the morning and exercise. It's what's keeping me alive." Despite gaining back some weight, Delores says, "I've never been healthier in my life. I've lowered my blood pressure medicine a bunch. It's been three years [since diagnosis] and I haven't been sick a day. I don't even have headaches any more. Diabetes forces you to do what you should have done in the first place." ▪

"I CAN GO TO THE GYM AND WORK IT OFF."

Graduating from college, landing that first job, moving from student life to full-time work—times of transition can make staying with an exercise routine difficult.

For recent college graduate Sara Martin, 23, exercising with a friend helps her stay with the program. Recently, they decided to join a health club. "We found it harder to exercise regularly in the summer," says Sara. They might make occasional tennis dates, but it was too easy to bag it. If it was hard to stick with it when the weather was good, winter might prove impossible. Sara felt joining a club would help. Making a financial commitment can be an incentive, too, she found. "You paid the money, you might as well go. I use it for motivation," she says. Plus, she knew how much she enjoyed working out in a club. She can easily vary her workout—sometimes opting for a step aerobics class, other times joining a high-impact aerobics session, or using state-of-the-art equipment like stairclimbing machines or weights.

Sara's had insulin-dependent diabetes for 11 years. Although she does not have a formal exercise prescription, she says her doctor has always emphasized the benefits of regular exercise. Staying active is something that's been second nature to Sara. During her years at Marymount College in Arlington, Virginia, she worked out at in the campus gym, walked, or went running.

Now with a full-time job, she's still determined to make time for fitness. She exercises in the evenings after dinner. "I go to the gym probably five times a week," she says. Three times a week, she does an hour of aerobics in a class. The other two days she'll work out on the stairclimber and go through a weight routine. Her only exercise goal: staying fit.

But, Sara's found a fringe benefit: regular workouts provide stress release. "It's good to know when I'm going to go [to the gym] every day. It's something to look forward to. If I'm at work and I have a really bad day, I can go the gym and work it off." ▪

weight, count on exercising five times a week. Consider that exercise can be a great way to accomplish two things at once. For example, you can read or watch television while riding a stationary bicycle. You might also use a family group sporting activity as a way to spend fun time together.

Can you afford it? This is an important consideration. Some exercise activities can be expensive. Many forms of exercise require a small, possibly one-time investment. Others require a bigger one, such as ongoing dues or monthly payments. Take a realistic look at your budget and plan accordingly. Unfortunately, when finances get tight, it's often the exercise club that gets cut out first. Because money can be a motivator, some athletic clubs ask that you agree to 12 months of automatic payments when you sign up. The thinking is that if you are paying for it, you might as well use it. It also gives you a year to make some positive changes in your lifestyle.

Do you have a good support network? One of the most effective ways to help maintain your motivation is to share an activity with other people. It also helps to have the support of friends and family.

Conversely, one of the quickest ways to get discouraged and lose your mental momentum to exercise is to have a friend or family member dampen your spirits. Some friends or family members might be jealous of your resolve to exercise and offer pessimistic comments. Some family members might resent you being away while you exercise. Maybe they don't like the times that you've chosen to exercise and will try to discourage you from going. They may even laugh at you.

Having the support of family and friends can help you keep with it. If there are conflicts, try to resolve them.

Explain to the critics that you need their support and ask them to hold their criticism until you see some results.

It will also help to surround yourself with people you know who are going through similar challenges. Associate with people who exercise regularly and share experiences with them. Read exercise literature to help keep you charged up.

STICKING WITH IT

You'll need to keep up your new, more active lifestyle for several months before it becomes a natural part of your life. Exercising for good health is a life-long pursuit. Like other pursuits that bring you joy, you will reach a time when you really miss exercising if you have to stop for a little while because of travel, special events, or illness.

If you're serious about sticking with your exercise program, here are some strategies that may work for you.

Set a schedule and keep it.

Make your exercise schedule in advance. We all live busy lives, so take out your calendar and pencil in the times that you will exercise. Make the commitment to exercise just as you would any other important appointment. But be realistic: the time should be convenient so that you have no excuses not to change your clothes and work out. Remember, habits are developed through practice. And your hard-won fitness can be lost quickly when you neglect it.

To increase your chances for success, ask yourself

■ Am I scheduling exercise at times when I am free from other duties? For instance, will someone else watch the kids or will anyone mind if we eat later on some days?

- Am I allowing myself enough time to change and shower afterward so that I can meet the rest of my schedule?
- Will I really get up early three days a week to exercise, or should I plan to work out in the afternoon or at night?
- Will I be able to stick to this schedule each week?

It helps to schedule your exercise at the same times each week so that you develop the habit. In addition, a set pattern will also help you to adapt your diabetes control more successfully, especially when you're just starting out. If you do the same exercise at the same time on the same days, by testing your blood, you'll begin to know what effect exercise has on your blood glucose level. Once you have this knowledge, you can begin to experiment with other exercises at new times.

Get a training partner.

Consider the benefits of exercising with someone else. We all have days when we are easily tempted to skip our workout. Chances are, however, that your training partner will be strong on a day that you are weak and be ready to go before you can change your mind. It's also important to be strong for your partner, too. Training with someone can be a lot of fun. You'll have someone with whom to talk and to share experiences.

When you choose a partner, find someone who is committed to sticking with it. It helps if you have similar goals. Consider someone who is in about the same physical condition you are. Someone who is really fit might tempt you to exercise at their level, causing you to push too hard for safe exercise.

A training partner who knows about your diabetes can keep your exercise sessions even safer for you.

Cross-train.

Doing the same thing every time you exercise can get boring. It's also a good idea to have an alternate form of exercise available to you in case you get injured, for when the weather is bad, or for when you are traveling.

Many people alternate exercises daily. It's called cross-training. This is a method in which you alternate between different forms of exercise to prevent putting a specific strain on a particular part of the body day after day. In other words, you might ride a bicycle one day, walk the next, and swim another day. Cross-training is good for motivation because it gives you variety. It reduces the risk for injuries by letting your body rest and repair between sessions using the same muscles.

Set goals.

"If you fail to plan, you plan to fail," is an old adage but one with a lot of truth in it. Setting specific goals for yourself and then evaluating how you are doing with your goals is a great way to keep on track. But goals can work against you, too. If you set a goal that is not quickly attainable, you might get discouraged when you don't see immediate progress. Like Rome, your healthier body can't be built in a day!

Let's say one of your goals is to lose 30 pounds. First, you need to make the goal specific—set the date when you want to be 30 pounds lighter. Second, cut this big goal down into manageable chunks—set the date when you want to have lost the first 10 pounds. As anyone who has tried to lose weight knows, taking off 30 pounds will take a lot of time and patience—even if you exercise seven days a week!

This approach means you must set two goals: a short-term goal and a long-term goal. Let's start with your long-term goal—to lose 30 pounds. Determine realistically how long it will take you to lose that weight. You won't be able to lose it in a month. Maybe you think you can do it within 12 months. For most motivated people, this is probably realistic.

Now you can switch your focus to short-term goals. How much weight must you lose each month to work steadily toward your long-term goal? In this example, that's just 2 and a half pounds each month—very realistic.

Will you weigh yourself every week or every month? Will you allow yourself to lose extra weight one month to make up for the weight that didn't come off the month before? Figure out what your rules are, and seal the agreement with yourself.

Because life is full of surprises, some weeks and months will be better than others. But consider this: the slower and steadier your weight loss, the more likely it is that the weight won't be gained right back. Worthwhile projects take time. Keep reminding yourself of your goals and why you want to reach them. If you repeatedly miss reaching your short-term goals, you may not have been realistic when setting your goals. Rethink them and set new ones.

Failure versus backsliding.

Some people set themselves up for failure by ignoring their successes. Does the following sound familiar? You tell yourself that you aren't doing well enough. Then, when you have to miss several days of working out or you don't meet your expectations, you feel like you've failed. You forget to focus on the successes you've had during other weeks and months.

It is important to understand that you will have "off" days in any long-term exercise program. This is called backsliding. When you do, it is not because you have failed. You are just having an off day. Even the most dedicated, world-class athletes have off days. When you have an off day, assure yourself that it is simply a temporary backslide and that you will get back on track today. Then, make it happen. Forgive yourself for a little backsliding, and put it behind you.

Reward yourself.

One good way to keep your motivation high is to reward yourself when you accomplish a goal. For example, decide that if you meet this month's goal, you will reward yourself with some new clothes, a new book, a compact disc—anything that will help you stay committed. A good strategy is to set small rewards to the small goals that you set and bigger rewards for real milestones that you reach. Another hint: don't use food as a reward. ❧

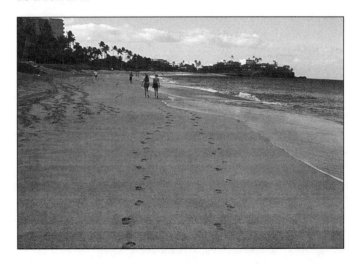

Dance, dance,
for the figure is easy,
the tune is catching
and will not stop.
Dance till the stars
come down from
the rafters.
Dance, dance, dance
till you drop.
—W.H. Auden

Getting Your *Body* Ready to Exercise

WHAT'S THE BEST WAY TO MAKE SURE YOUR EXERCISE PROGRAM IS TAILORED TO YOUR PARTICULAR NEEDS? Have a thorough medical examination before you begin. For each of us, the benefits of exercise must outweigh the risks. That means we need to know our health status. This knowledge gives us confidence to work out within our limits.

A thorough preexercise examination and fitness testing

should give you the following information:

- Your blood pressure
- Your blood fat levels
- The health of your heart and circulatory system
- Your body composition, fat versus lean
- Your chances for bringing on or worsening diabetes complications, and
- Your appropriate exercise level.

YOUR PREEXERCISE PHYSICAL

Before you make the appointment with your doctor to discuss beginning an exercise program, think about your goals. Do you want to lose weight? Do you want to have more strength and energy for your daily life? Do you want to lower your blood glucose levels? Do you want to stay fit despite your recent diagnosis? Do you want to avoid specific diabetes complications?

You will also want to think about how your diabetes care might keep you from reaching your goals. Your doctor can measure your blood fat levels and assess how well your heart is working, but he or she will need to learn from you how diabetes affects your day-to-day life and behavior. Do you often have mysterious high blood glucose readings? Are you puzzled by numbness, coldness, or tingling in your hands or feet? Do you have frequent hypoglycemia? Are you able to sense hypoglycemia before your blood glucose level becomes very low? Has a recent weight gain got you anxious?

By the time you have finished with your preexercise physical exam and fitness testing, you should be able to complete a chart of exercise goals (Table 1).

Your personal health history.

Ask your doctor to work with you to obtain a complete medical history and to understand your individual resources and lifestyle preferences. Be sure to mention anything about your health that's troubling you. Good communication with your doctor is one key to keeping your health the best it can be. If you tend to "blank out" during your office visits, write a list of questions and concerns ahead of time, and don't be shy about reading it while you're talking with your doctor.

First, here's a basic question: do you have type I or type II diabetes? If you are not sure, ask your doctor. You may be confused because:

- People over 30 years old can develop type I diabetes.
- People under 30 can develop type II diabetes.
- Some people with type II diabetes require insulin injections.

The doctor will look at your ability to make insulin (people with type I diabetes eventually lose the ability to make insulin) and your tendency to make high levels of ketones (ketosis is much more common in type I diabetes) when deciding what type of diabetes you have.

List for your doctor all of the medications, prescription or over-the-counter, that you take. This list could include heart and blood pressure pills, thyroid medication, eye drops for glaucoma, drugs for asthma, or headache remedies. Almost any drug has the potential to affect your ability to exercise.

Your blood glucose control will also be very important. Don't forget to bring in your self-monitoring records. Your doctor will attempt to develop an appropriate strategy to avoid or minimize any blood glucose problems you may encounter with exercise.

Because you have diabetes, you are at risk for heart and blood vessel disease. Do you have additional risk factors, such as cigarette smoking, a family history of heart trouble, cholesterol or triglyceride abnormalities, and blood pressure problems? Your doctor will look for symptoms of existing heart and blood vessel disease. Have you noticed chest pain or discomfort that comes on with exertion like carrying groceries or climbing stairs? Often people describe this as a squeezing pain or tightness in the chest that may spread to the shoulder or jaw. Pain is caused by inadequate blood flow to the heart. It may or may not be associated with nausea, hiccups, sweating, shortness of breath, heart pounding, or even gas, bloating, or gastrointestinal distress. This discomfort, called angina, is an important indication of significant heart disease. It can be treated. In diabetes, nerve damage may keep you from feeling these symptoms. This is why an electrocardiogram is an important preexercise test.

Are you bothered by leg pains or cramps (most often in the calves) while walking or during exercise that go away when you rest? This is due to a brief lack of blood flow to the muscles, called *intermittent claudication*. It can be treated.

Another potential problem is a temporary blockage of blood flow to the brain. This may result in momentary episodes of dizziness, loss of vision, or weakness or numbness in a specific area of the body. If you have any of these symptoms, be sure to discuss them with your doctor. Dizziness after standing up quickly can also be due to low blood pressure.

Your doctor will look for nerve damage, which is particularly common in the feet and hands of people with diabetes. Damage to the sensory nerves of your foot can cause loss of sensation. This can affect your ability to feel an injury or judge the fit of your exercise shoes, so make sure your doctor tests it. Let your doctor know if you have problems keeping your balance. Nerve damage can also affect the involuntary control of your heart rate, sweating, and blood pressure.

Looking into your body.

The next steps in your exam are laboratory tests and a physical. Take a deep breath, relax, and have your blood pressure checked. Depending on how long you've had diabetes and what shape your body was in when you were diagnosed, your doctor will check for evidence of the long-term complications of diabetes affecting the heart, blood vessels, eyes, kidneys, and nerves. One kind of blood test, which measures glycated hemoglobin, will show how well you have been controlling your diabetes. This test gives a kind of average of blood glucose control by measuring how much glucose is attached to hemoglobin, a part of the red blood cell. More glucose attaches to the hemoglobin when blood glucose levels are high than when they are are low. Other blood tests can be used to evaluate your risks for heart disease (cholesterol and triglycerides) and to look for any abnormalities that might interfere with your ability to exercise (infection, thyroid function, anemia). Table 2 gives values for some of these blood tests. You may be asked to collect urine for 24 hours to assess your kidney function.

The doctor will listen to your heart and lungs. If indicated, your doctor will hook you up for an electrocardiogram, a tracing of your heart's electrical activity, while you are lying down. This will show any unusual patterns in how your heart is working, such as a heart rate that does not increase during exercise. If you are older than 35 or have developed any long-term com-

TABLE 1

My Preexercise Health Status And Goals

Date: _____ Starting Body Weight: _____

Aerobic Capacity: _____ Body Composition: _____

Fasting Blood Glucose: _____ Glycated Hemoglobin: _____

Resting Heart Rate: _____ Resting Blood Pressure: _____

Total Cholesterol: _____ LDL Cholesterol: _____

HDL Cholesterol: _____ Triglycerides: _____

Waist Measurement: _____ Hip Measurement: _____

Waist/Hip Ratio: _____

Long-Term Goal: _____

_____

Short-Term Goals:

_____

_____

_____

_____

TABLE 2
VALUES FOR COMMON BLOOD TESTS
(VALUES IN MG/DL EXCEPT HEMOGLOBIN)

	Normal (nondiabetic)	Goal	Acceptable	Poor
Fasting or premeal blood glucose	<115	<120	120–140	>140
Postmeal blood glucose	<140	<180	180–220	>220
Glycated hemoglobin*	<7%	<8%	<9%	≥9%
Total cholesterol	<200	<200	200–240	>240
LDL cholesterol	<130	<130	130–159	≥160
HDL cholesterol	—	—	—	≤35
Triglycerides	<150	<200	200–399	≥400

*Ask your doctor to help you adjust this according to the type of test that is done for your doctor.

Adapted from *Medical Management of Type II Diabetes Mellitus.* Alexandria, VA, Am. Diabetes Assoc., 1994

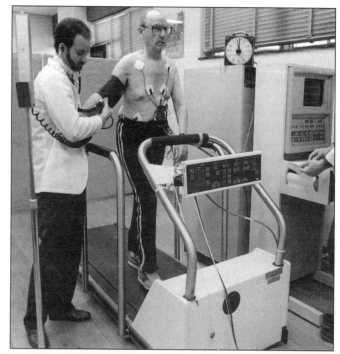

The purpose of the treadmill test is to find out how much exercise you can do. Blood pressure, electrocardiogram, and heart rate are measured throughout the test.
Photograph by Kent Miller, courtesy of Indiana University Adult Fitness Program.

plications or if your doctor is unsatisfied with the results of your electrocardiogram, you may be asked to get an exercise stress test (see below).

Your doctor should examine how well your nervous system is working. He or she will test your reflexes, your sense of touch, and your ability to feel where your body parts are in relation to your surroundings. You may have tests looking at how your heart responds to slow deep breathing or to holding your breath and pushing forcefully. Your doctor may also check to see how your blood pressure reacts when you sit down or when you stand up after lying down.

Make sure your doctor examines your feet for callouses, corns, blisters, deformities, or evidence of inflammation or infections like athlete's foot. Get specific instructions from the doctor on how you should care for any of these when they occur.

Other specialists.

Some of your test results may show that you need to visit a specialist, such as a cardiologist, ophthalmologist, or neurologist. At the very least, you need an eye examination before beginning to exercise. This is vital to your sight if you have already been told you have retinopathy. Depending on your overall fitness, some forms of exercise may put your eyesight at risk and may need to be crossed off your list.

A diet history and an exercise history are two other important parts of your preexercise assessment. A dietitian will need to get an idea of your current food plan, including eating patterns and preferences, so that recommendations can be made to accommodate or enhance your exercise program. An exercise physiologist or other exercise specialist may ask you questions about your current level of activity as well as when, where, and how you would most like to exercise.

If all this activity makes you feel as though you are preparing for something big, you're right! Changing your life to bring more enjoyment into it is a significant decision and needs proper preparation.

EXERCISE TESTING

Exercise testing usually involves several types of measurements. Your weight, height, and blood pressure and an exercise stress test are usually standard features of exercise testing. In addition, you may have your body composition determined by an assessment of amount of body fat. You may be given a test to determine your flexibility.

Exercise stress test.

It takes energy to exercise. Muscles require oxygen to get energy from the foods we eat. The harder you exercise, the more oxygen you will have to use. Oxygen is delivered to the muscles by the lungs, the heart, and the blood vessels. Muscles that are unaccustomed to physical activity may be unable to take enough oxygen out of the blood during exercise and may tire faster than muscles that have been trained. The more fit you are, the more oxygen you can consume, and the more exercise you will be able to do.

Your ability to use oxygen as well as the responses of your muscles, heart, lungs, and blood vessels can be measured during an exercise stress test. It may be done while you are riding a stationary bicycle or walking on a treadmill. Electrodes will be placed on your chest so that a tracing of the electrical activity of your heart can be made. Blood pressure will also be monitored by a blood pressure cuff on your arm. You will be asked to exercise for a certain length of time or possibly until you can't go any further.

During exercise, blood pressure changes. If you have high blood pressure, or are likely to develop high blood pressure, your pressure may rise excessively with exercise. If you have heart disease, irregular heart beats or changes in the electrocardiogram may develop as the heart works harder to supply oxygen and nutrients to the exercising muscles. This test will allow your doctor to monitor you while you exercise under very safe, controlled conditions. It can provide valuable information about health factors that may limit your ability to exercise and can help determine your level of physical fitness.

When the test begins, you will be exercising at a

TABLE 3

VALUES FOR VO$_2$ MAX MEASUREMENT TO DETERMINE AEROBIC CAPACITY

Age:	20s	30s	40s	50s	60+
WOMEN					
Excellent	>36.9	>35.6	>32.8	>31.4	>30.2
Good	33.0–36.9	31.5–35.6	29.0–32.8	27.0–31.4	24.5–30.2
Average	29.0–32.9	27.0–31.4	24.5–28.9	22.8–26.9	20.2–24.4
Poor	<29.0	<27.0	<24.5	<22.8	<20.2
MEN					
Excellent	>46.4	>44.9	>43.7	>40.9	>36.4
Good	42.5–46.4	41.0–44.9	39.0–43.7	35.8–40.9	32.2–36.4
Average	36.5–42.4	35.5–40.9	33.6–38.9	31.0–35.7	26.1–32.2
Poor	<36.5	<35.5	<33.6	<31.0	<26.1

Adapted from Cooper KH: *The Aerobics Way*. New York, Bantam, 1977

a mouthpiece or into a mask worn over your mouth. You will reach your limit for exercise when your body reaches its maximum level for consuming oxygen. This measurement, known as your aerobic (with oxygen) capacity or VO$_2$ max, tells how fit your heart and lungs are. Your VO$_2$ max is used to select an appropriate exercise intensity. Table 3 gives values for VO$_2$ max.

If abnormalities show up during the test, you may be sent for further evaluation for heart disease or you may be given medications to control problems like high blood pressure. One long-term complication of diabetes, a type of autonomic neuropathy, is damage to the nerves that sense pain in the heart. The exercise test may show significant heart trouble before you develop symptoms of heart disease, such as chest pain or shortness of breath. After these potential problems are identified and treated if necessary, an exercise prescription can be developed to ensure that you are exercising at a level that is safe and effective.

How flexible are you?

If increased range of movement is one of your fitness goals, you will want to mark your progress by having your flexibility measured. There is no one test for overall flexibility. Each test is specific to the joints being tested. There are tests to measure the flexibility of the

slow, comfortable pace. The difficulty or intensity of exercise will be gradually increased. The slope of the treadmill may be increased (so you walk uphill) or the resistance on the bicycle may be adjusted so it takes more force to pedal. You will keep at it until fatigue occurs or abnormalities appear with your blood pressure or in your heart tracing. The length of time of exercise varies from a few minutes to as long as 20 minutes.

The more exercise you can do, the more oxygen you will use. Your consumption of oxygen may be measured during the test by having you breathe out through

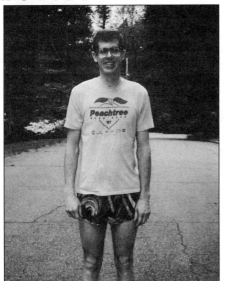

"RUNNING MAKES ME FEEL GOOD." For Tom Pogue, running wasn't always fun. It was more like pure drudgery. He wasn't consistent and wouldn't stick to the running, which he says made it harder because he kept having to go through that initial difficult period. One tactic he used with some success was to sign up for races so he would have to run to get ready for them. "Plus," says Tom, "I love to eat, and running helps keep my weight from ballooning."

Once he could run three miles comfortably, he started enjoying it. Now Tom is in the habit of running between 15 and 20 miles a week—3 to 4 miles on three weekday mornings and a longer run, around 6 miles, on a weekend morning. He found it fun to occasionally run longer distances, and he has completed half and full marathons. "Training for a marathon will teach you things about your body," he says. In Tom's case, pain in his knees and back led him to a podiatrist, who fitted Tom with orthotics (small pads to redistribute weight) for his running shoes.

Tom was an experienced runner when the diagnosis of type I diabetes at age 32 threw him off stride. "Diabetes made me look at everything I do in a different light. I had to think about 'when' and 'how' I did everything. Running was no exception. I was a little apprehensive." Luckily, Tom's endocrinologist, a runner himself, encouraged Tom to keep running. He's been careful to look at the effects running has had on Tom's blood glucose level and has given Tom specific suggestions on how to adjust his insulin routine for running in general and for longer races in particular.

After starting insulin, Tom was referred to a diabetes education program at a hospital, and he signed up for sessions on specific topics, exercise among them. Some of the advice wasn't too practical. "I was told that the ideal time to exercise was one hour after eating, to lessen the chances of an insulin reaction—but that's the last time I want to run, on a full stomach." In addition, Tom was advised to test his blood glucose before and after running, but with his doctor's approval, he discarded this "one-size-fits-all" approach to diabetes and exercise and only tests before he starts. (In all, Tom tests four or five times a day.)

By self-monitoring frequently, Tom is able to individualize his diabetes management. He controls his blood glucose levels with four insulin injections a day. His routine is to run first thing in the morning. He tests first, then runs, and injects his insulin and eats when he's back home. If his pre-run glucose test results are low, he has a glass of orange juice before he starts out. A few times, he has had mild insulin reactions while running, usually when he runs later in the day, after his morning insulin injection. Tom says, "It's mainly a fuzzy-headed feeling but still not the way you want to feel when you are finishing a hard run." Tom carries glucose tablets and an extra quarter or two in a pocket he weaves through his shoe laces. He has also learned that he should inject into his abdomen before running—injecting in his thigh before running speeded up his absorption of insulin and led to reactions.

Through trial and error, Tom developed a plan to keep running, even with diabetes. He's happy with what he's learned. He says, "It's tempting not to vary your routine at all to avoid problems, but I've had enough experiences by now to be more willing to try new things." New things like the Boston Marathon, perhaps.

Tom is convinced that running helps him control diabetes. "My doctor tells me I take about one-third less insulin each day than someone of the same weight would take. I can tell how much running helps my control when I have to stop for up to a week because of a cold—by the end of the week, my blood glucose levels are much more erratic than usual. Besides, running makes me feel good. I get charged up!" ■

TABLE 4

VALUES (IN INCHES) FOR THE SIT-AND-REACH TEST TO DETERMINE FLEXIBILITY

Age:	20s	30s	40s	50s	60+
WOMEN					
Excellent	>24	>23	>22	>21	>20
Good	22–23	21–22	20–21	19–20	18–19
Average	16–21	15–20	14–19	13–18	12–17
Poor	<12	<11	<10	<9	<8
MEN					
Excellent	>22	>21	>20	>19	>18
Good	19–21	18–20	17–19	16–18	15–17
Average	13–18	12–17	11–16	10–15	9–14
Poor	<9	<8	<7	<6	<5

Adapted from Golding LA, Myers CR, Sinning WE (Eds.): *The Y's Way to Physical Fitness*. Rosemont, IL, Young Mens' Christian Assoc., USA, 1982

back, legs, hips, shoulders, ankle, and the upper body (trunk). Before being tested, make sure you warm up a little and do some stretches.

The most common method for measuring flexibility is the sit-and-reach test. It measures the amount of flexibility you have in your lower back and backs of the legs (hamstrings). In this test, you sit on the floor with your legs straight in front and your feet about 10 to 12 inches apart. A line is drawn from heel to heel, and a yardstick is placed between your legs with the 0-mark end closest to your hips and the 15-inch mark at the heel line. With your arms extended in front of you and one hand on top of the other, you bend forward at the hips. Slowly and without bouncing, you reach along the yardstick as far forward as you can and hold the position for at least 1 second. Table 4 gives some standard values for the sit-and-reach test. These numbers show how far down the yardstick your fingers reach.

How much of your body is fat?

We usually think of body fat as something bad, but everybody needs some fat. Fat serves as a supply of energy for basic body processes. However, having too much body fat is unhealthy. To be fit, you need to have a healthy proportion of muscle and other lean body tissues and fat. Muscle is important in improving the levels of high-density lipoprotein cholesterol (the good cholesterol) while reducing triglycerides, a type of blood fat that promotes atherosclerosis or hardening of the arteries. Too much fat, on the other hand, increases insulin resistance, contributing to hard-to-control blood glucose levels. Being overfat also makes people more likely to have high blood pressure. Carrying around a lot of extra fat also increases your bulk, making your heart work harder without adding to your ability to move. For these reasons, body composition is an important part of fitness. Body composition tests measure how much fat you have compared to the portion of your body that is lean or fat free.

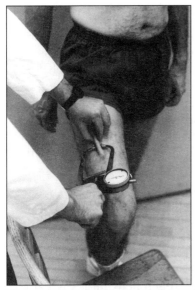
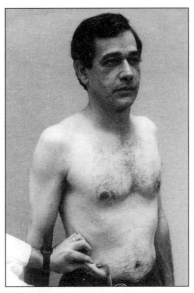

Two common sites for measuring skinfold thickness.
Photographs by Kevin Hutchinson, courtesy of Indiana University Adult Fitness Program.

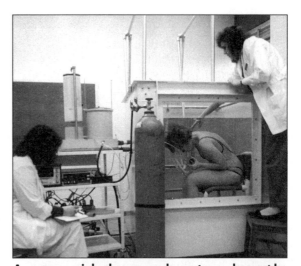

A person weighed on an underwater scale must be totally submerged. Body fat is estimated by comparing weight under water to weight out of water.
Photograph by Kent Miller, courtesy of Indiana University Adult Fitness Program.

Although just being weighed and measured for height will estimate the body fat, there are more precise methods. The scales alone can't tell the whole story. For example, if a 250-pound body builder with rippling muscles is compared to an average person of similar height and weight, the weight lifter would have less fat.

Women generally have a greater percentage of body fat than men. The amount of body fat you have is measured as a percentage of total components. For instance, healthy, normal-weight women usually have between 23 and 28 percent body fat. This means that lean or fat-free components—bones, muscles, and water—make up the other 72 to 77 percent of the body. Healthy men usually have 15 to 20 percent body fat. For

comparison, female athletes may have less than 15 percent body fat, and male athletes may have less than 10 percent body fat.

A simple way to estimate the amount of body fat you have is to have someone take thickness measurements of the fat on several areas of your body. This is called a skinfold test. A person trained in the use of calipers will gently pinch a fold of skin between the ends of the calipers and use the numbers to calculate total fat. The upper arm, hip, abdomen, thigh, upper back, or chest are all commonly used sites for this estimate. The accuracy of the measurement will depend directly on the amount of experience and training your measurer has had. The measurements are then put into an equation, which results in an estimate of overall body fat.

A more accurate way to estimate total body fat is hydrostatic or underwater weighing. First, you are weighed on a standard scale and then you are weighed under water. Because fat floats, a person with a large amount of fat will weigh less underwater than another person of the same size with less fat. The difference in the two weights is used to create an estimate of your body density, from which an estimate of amount of body fat can be made. A lot of wellness centers and universities and some fitness clubs have facilities for underwater weighing. To increase the accuracy of the results, the amount of air remaining in the lungs must be accounted for. Also, your results should be specific for your age and gender, because bone density plays a part in how much you weigh.

Some athletic clubs and medical programs estimate body fat with light. This is called infrared interactance, and it uses the fact that fat bends light differently than does protein or water. A beam of light is directed into the biceps muscle of the upper arm; the light scatters according to how much body fat is in the tissue above the muscle. The scatter can be used to estimate the amount of body fat. The technique of the measurer generally does not affect the results. But, because the scattering pattern of just one muscle is used, it's inaccurate for judging total body fat.

Another way to estimate the total amount of body fat is to run a gentle electrical current through the body and measure how fast it goes from one point to another. This method is based on the fact that water, muscle, and bone let electricity pass through much faster than does fat, which tends to slow down the current. Fat acts as an insulator that resists the electrical flow. When resistance is measured in various parts of the body, the amount of fat can be estimated. The drawback is that some people have a larger proportion of water in their body than others. For people with diabetes, poor blood glucose control can lead to inaccurate results. When blood glucose is high, you can be over- or under-hydrated, depending on how long you've been hyperglycemic. Wait until your blood glucose level is within your target range to have this test.

Where's your fat?

The total amount of body fat is meaningful, but the location of that fat may play an even more important role. Fat that is mainly in the abdominal area and upper body (known as an apple-shaped fat distribution) comes with a higher risk for disease than fat found over the hips and thighs (pear-shaped fat distribution). For some reason, upper-body fat cells are larger and more insulin resistant than lower-body fat cells.

The tendency to deposit more fat in one area than another is in part inherited. However, those who smoke are more prone to have abdominal obesity, whether or not they are obese.

After overall body fat is estimated by skinfold thickness, you can use these measurements to determine your fat distribution. Divide the skinfold measurement of your upper back by the measurement of your upper arm. If the result equals more than 1, you carry your fat on the upper body.

An additional way to look at your body fat distribution is to compare your waist measurement with your hip measurement. Measure each in inches with a tape measure. Then divide your waist measurement by your hip measurement. A result greater than 1 for men or

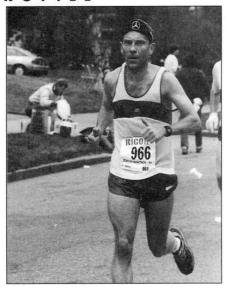

"YOU HAVE TO COUNT ON YOURSELF."

At 38, John Madden, Jr., is a veteran marathoner. Since running his first marathon in 1978, he's completed 12 races. Perhaps the standout among them, the 1991 Leningrad [St. Petersburg] "Biele Noche" or "White Nights" Marathon, held on June 22, the summer solstice and longest day of the year. On this day, the city has about 21 hours of sunlight and the remaining hours are bathed in what Madden terms, "an eerie twilight." With night turned into day, the White Nights race begins at 11 p.m. The 26.2-mile race begins and ends in Leningrad's historic Palace Square.

For Madden, the race was more than an opportunity to experience Glasnost first hand. Finishing in 2:48:45, a personal best, he qualified as the first American finisher. Madden's visit, as part of a tour group of American runners, was also a chance to meet Russian runners. He'd heard that running shoes were in short supply in the Soviet Union. "I brought used running shoes. They don't have any running shoe factories, so people are running in barefeet and in street shoes. We met a group of runners and had a lovely tea in this huge Stalinist gym. We all brought three or four pairs of old running shoes, and they were all salivating for these shoes that no amount of money they could save could buy."

Madden is also a veteran of living with type I diabetes. John was diagnosed after a bout with the flu. He was 14. His younger brother was diagnosed at the same time. While the boys were hospitalized, Madden remembers a visitor who made a difference. "We got a visit from Bill Talbert. He was a friend of a friend. He didn't know us at all. It was within a few days of our being diagnosed, and it made a big impression. Here was someone who had dealt with it very well, that early on was a good example." (Tennis great Bill Talbert was diagnosed with diabetes in the 1928, at the age of 10. In the 1940s and 1950s, Bill racked up 38 tennis titles. In 1946, he and partner Gardnar Mulloy were the first men's doubles team to win the U.S. Open three times. By 1950, Bill was ranked number two player at Wimbledon. From 1953 to 1957, he captained the U.S. Davis Cup Team, and for 15 years served as director of the U.S. Open Tennis Championships in Forest Hills, New York.)

Both John and his brother went on to run track in high school. John remembers that less than six months after diagnosis he was on the cross-country team. "I won every race that year, and I broke the school record, and I was a sophomore. It was an ecstatic feeling."

Did diabetes ever interfere with his running? "No. I think people like the track team coaches and so on probably didn't really know what to think in terms of what support I might need. I was very independent. That's one thing you learn very early when you have diabetes. You have to count on yourself to see that you're all right. But I never had any problems in competition, because I would make sure to eat something beforehand."

Remembering those days, John also recalls having to rely on urine testing for blood glucose levels. "I shudder to think of making adjustments to insulin based on that."

Today, John relies heavily on blood glucose testing. "I test very frequently. I suppose someone newly diagnosed with diabetes might say it's a pain, but it gives you great freedom. It doesn't restrict you in any way. Without testing you'd be in the dark. You'd be ignorant. It doesn't take any time. It's not painful, and it's highly informative. Information makes you free."

After a hiatus from running during college, John began working out regularly during law school. An attorney in Manhattan, he usually runs in the evenings after work in New York City. In terms of distance running and his diabetes regimen, John says he learned a lot from trial and error. His current physician is supportive of marathoning and distance running. John adds that "I have found as a general principle that diabetics—athletes or not—have to learn from their own experience. Yes, obviously listen to what your doctor says, but you're more responsible than the doctor [for your self-care]. I think perhaps older people with type II diabetes are more apt to put great faith in doctors. That lays off the responsibility on someone else, and people with diabetes must take care of themselves."

Part of Madden's routine is keeping a log of his runs and his mileage. He aims for one long run per week. At least one day a week he does a nonrunning workout, such as working out on a stairclimber, to cut back on the pounding and stress of running on city streets.

Still, nothing is quite a satisfying as getting in a good run. "I like running because I like looking at things in New York. It's active rather than passive. I like running through different neighborhoods and seeing what's going on. I like that as well as competing. Competing isn't the only reason to exercise. If competition was the only thing that motivated me, I'd have stopped." ■

greater than 0.8 for women is considered an indication that more body fat is carried on the upper body than the lower body.

Who does exercise testing?

If your doctor does not perform exercise testing, ask your doctor or your health-care delivery system for a referral to an exercise physiologist or a wellness program that does exercise testing. Many universities with health centers have wellness programs for people with diabetes or heart disease. Wellness programs offer fitness testing by exercise physiologists who will work with your doctor to write an exercise prescription that's just for you. You might consider traveling to a wellness program for a short stay to get you on the right track. ❧

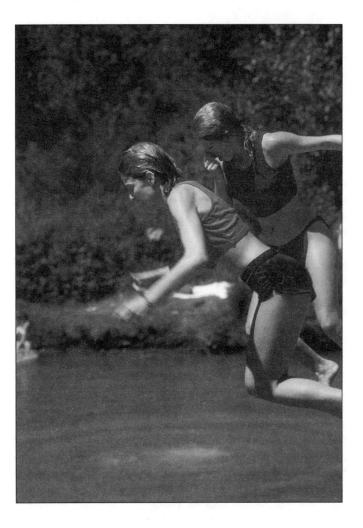

Do you know that old age may come after you with equal grace, force, and fascination?

—Walt Whitman

Your *Exercise* Prescription

ONCE YOU HAVE COMPLETED YOUR PRE-EXERCISE PHYSICAL AND EXERCISE TESTS, WHAT SHOULD YOU DO? How hard should you exercise? How long? How often? Where do you start? Hopefully, either your doctor or an exercise physiologist or another health-care professional recommended by your doctor can help you develop an exercise plan that suits your likes and dislikes and meets your goals. There is no standard formula. The type of exercise you do, the intensity, duration, frequency, and way you progress should all be planned with you in mind.

The results you get from an exercise program are determined by two important principles of exercise training. The principle of specificity tells us that any change in fitness will be specific to those systems and parts of the body that are exercised and the way in which they are exercised. For example, the oxygen-consuming (aerobic) system of the body is improved by activities that cause an increase in heart rate and breathing as more and more oxygen is delivered specifically to the muscles you use during the exercise. Do not expect aerobic activities for your legs to increase aerobic fitness in the muscles of your arms or to improve the strength or flexibility of your legs.

The overload principle tells us that the body must work over and above what it normally does to bring about improvements. The work of exercise must be hard enough to boost fitness without causing unreasonable stress. The amount of work actually needed to increase fitness will be determined by the intensity (how hard), the duration (how long), and the frequency (how often) of exercise.

The American Diabetes Association has developed general guidelines for exercise for people with diabetes (Table 1). However, they are not specific to your needs and should be used only as an outline. Your exercise program will yield the best results if you and your doctor write an individualized prescription for you.

T A B L E   1

AMERICAN DIABETES ASSOCIATION GUIDELINES FOR EXERCISE

General guidelines:
- Use proper footwear and protective equipment.
- Avoid exercise in extreme heat or cold.
- Inspect your feet daily and after exercise.
- Avoid exercising during periods of poor blood glucose control.

Specifically for those with type I (insulin-dependent) diabetes:
- Exercise is recommended to improve your cardiovascular fitness and psychological well-being and for social interaction and recreation. Safe participation in all forms of exercise, consistent with your lifestyle, should be the main goal. Participation in competitive sports is possible if you so desire. You need to self-monitor your blood glucose so that necessary adjustments can be made in diet or insulin dosage.

Specifically for those with type II (non-insulin-dependent) diabetes:
- Exercise should be part of your diabetes therapy, in addition to appropriate diet and medications, to improve your blood glucose control, reduce your risk of cardiovascular complications, and increase your psychological well-being. An exercise stress test is recommended if you are over 35 years of age. If you take oral hypoglycemic medications or insulin, you need to self-monitor your blood glucose level. Your exercise program should include moderate aerobic exercise (50–70% of VO_2 max) for 20–45 minutes at least 3 days per week. Always perform low-intensity warm-up and cool-down exercises.

WHAT SHOULD I DO?

The types of exercise you select should be based on the goals you have set, your level of fitness, any special safety considerations, the amount of time you have for exercise, availability of equipment and facilities, and your own personal likes and dislikes.

You should start by deciding just what you would like to get out of an exercise program. Think about the goals you chose before you had your preexercise exam. Do they still seem reasonable? Did your doctor agree that these goals were safe for you? Can you fill in the chart on exercise goals, found in Chapter 3?

You may need to discuss the goals you have in mind with other members of your health-care team. For instance, if your goal is to lose weight and you use insulin injections, both your doctor and your dietitian should work with you to set clear, achievable goals, because you will be making adjustments in your insulin and eating routines.

Make sure your goals are appropriate, realistic, and achievable. Both short-term and long-term goals should be identified. Then, develop a systematic plan that helps you keep on track. For more encouragement on goal setting and sticking with it, see Chapter 2.

Your goals should also be specific and measurable. They may focus on regular participation or on specific health or fitness objectives. For example, you may have as your long-term goal to "do 45 minutes of aerobic exercise 5 days per week." In the first two weeks, your short-term goal may simply be to "show up for an organized aerobic fitness class on Monday, Wednesday, and Friday." After a month or two you might concentrate on increasing the time you are active. You may have as your new goal to "work up to 20 minutes of continuous aerobic exercise."

If you have as your long-term goal to "lose 50 pounds," it would be best to set short-term goals like, "lose 1 pound each week," or "lose 5 pounds each month."

Your level of fitness and any safety concerns should also help you decide what activities are best for you. Walking is an excellent choice for many people with diabetes, but if you are in super shape, a running program may be more appropriate. If your feet and legs have long-term complications of diabetes, it may be best to try a swimming program. Types of exercise you can do despite physical limitations are described in further detail in Chapter 8. There are many things you can do to meet your goals, but whatever you choose, make sure it's something that you enjoy and that fits easily into your lifestyle.

Three groups of activities may help you reach specific health and fitness goals.

Aerobic activities.

These are recommended for people with type II diabetes because the benefits include increased fitness of the heart, lungs, and blood vessels, improved blood glucose control, and better weight management. They help you reduce your risk of cardiovascular problems. The potential for cardiovascular benefits of aerobic activities also make them an excellent choice for many people with type I diabetes.

To qualify as aerobic exercise, an activity must use the large muscles of the body in continuous, rhythmical, sustained movement. When done at an appropriate intensity and duration, brisk walking, swimming, cycling, aerobic dance, rowing, cross-country skiing,

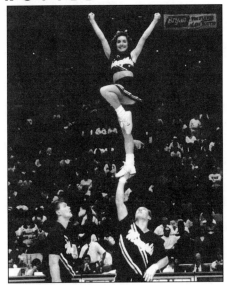

"I GREW UP EXERCISING."

You're watching college basketball on television. There's a break in the action and suddenly the screen pulsates with those impossibly energetic dynamos— college cheerleaders. The coed squad does tumbling runs, "stunts," and then forms a human pyramid. The crowd roars. The pyramid topples. Then it's back to the game.

If you had been watching a Memphis State game a few years ago, you would have seen Stephen Grooms. Grooms, a senior in 1993, was on the varsity cheerleading squad all four years.

If you're thinking collegiate cheerleading is some sort of lightweight, made-for-TV sport, think again. Just try catching a 120-pound woman 50 times during a basketball game. Cheerleading stunts, as they are called, involve coed squads with the men catching women squad members as they plummet from shoulders, peel off from pyramids, and fly through the air in tumbling routines. Squad members lead cheers and also do tumbling runs.

Gymnastics was Stephen Grooms' first love. "As a kid I would do rolls (somersaults) anywhere there was room. Front rolls, back rolls. Anywhere. Even in the movie theater. Mom and Dad decided it was time to put me in a gymnastics program." Stephen was three years old.

For the next ten years, he competed seriously in gymnastics. "I grew up exercising and working out. I was in the gym four hours a day, for at least 10 years of my life."

At age 11, Stephen was diagnosed with insulin-dependent diabetes. But unlike many children with type I diabetes, he was not severely ill at the time. Because his mother also has insulin-dependent diabetes, she spotted his symptoms immediately. Diabetes did not interfere with his love of gymnastics. Stephen says his mother was very supportive. "She wanted me to do anything I wanted to," he says.

While Stephen stayed with gymnastics, by high school he was no longer going to meets. Instead, he attended a high school for the performing arts in Memphis and did gymnastics exhibitions.

It was a girl friend who got him into stunting for college cheerleading. The team training workouts include free weights two days a week for shoulders and legs and then practicing stunts for an hour or so three days a week.

Grooms says his control is good now, but he ran into some problems about two years ago. "I was running low quite a bit. I went to the doctor and he just put me on four shots a day. I have had great control [since then]."

Stephen tests before each injection and "anytime I feel anyway strange or awkward." He tests as often as five times a day.

In 1991, at the Universal Cheerleaders Association's (UCA) College Cheerleading and Dance Team National Championship in San Antonio, Stephen and a teammate ranked 5th in the Partner Stunt National Championship. These championships are broadcast on ESPN.

For Stephen, who is working on a BS degree in fitness/wellness, athletics is a way of life. He says he thinks he'd like to coach gymnastics one day. "I played baseball and football in high school. I've always really enjoyed being an athlete, and I look forward to helping others reach their athletic goals." ■

roller skating, ice skating, stairclimbing, and running can all be considered aerobic activities.

Resistance training.

This is a group of activities used to develop muscular strength and endurance. It includes exercises like weight lifting; using special resistance machines; stretching elastic bands, tubing, or springs; or performing simple calisthenic exercises like sit-ups and push-ups. Resistance training can make you stronger and give you more energy. It can help you look better, feel better, and work and play better. It can also protect against injuries and improve health.

The risks of resistance training are somewhat different than aerobic exercise, and you should check with your health-care team to make certain this activity is appropriate for you. Resistance training, if done properly, can be a useful addition to an aerobic fitness program. Injury prevention, increased muscle and decreased body fat, and better general health can be important to many people with diabetes. For athletes, resistance training is essential for top performance in sports that require strength, speed, power, or large muscle size.

Flexibility exercises.

These can give you increased freedom of movement, decreased stress and muscular tension, and reduced risk of injury. There are many stretches to help you move freely and without pain. Stretching is a gentle form of exercise that almost anyone can do. No matter how stiff, tight, or tense you may be, you can become more limber if you stretch correctly and regularly.

HOW HARD SHOULD I EXERCISE?

You should work hard enough during exercise to increase your fitness without pushing so hard that you expose yourself to unnecessary risks. The American Diabetes Association recommends moderate aerobic activity at 50% to 70% VO_2 max (maximum volume of oxygen consumption). This intensity level has been proven to be effective for most people, while also being safe and comfortable. To know your VO_2 max, you must have an exercise test.

Your "comfort zone" for aerobic activity depends primarily on how much you are taxing your individual limit for using oxygen—your VO_2 max. If you attempt to do exercise that demands more oxygen than your body is able to provide (exercise above your VO_2 max), it will be very strenuous and painful. You may be able to push yourself through the discomfort long enough to last for 30 to 90 seconds, but eventually your body will force you to slow down. Even at your VO_2 max, it is unlikely you will push yourself to exercise that hard for longer than 3 to 5 minutes, unless you are a competitive athlete. To get fit, you do not need to force yourself to exercise at this level.

The exercise intensity that is right for you will depend on several factors. An exercise stress test will tell you your VO_2 max so you'll know how hard you should exercise. If you are just beginning a conditioning program, it's a good idea to gradually ease into the exercise habit. It is better to start out at a low intensity and duration (such as 40% VO_2 max or lower, for even 5 or 10 minutes) and gradually increase as your fitness level and tolerance to exercise improves. If you are a well-trained competitive athlete with diabetes, it may be fine for you to train at 70% to 85% of your VO_2 max or even higher.

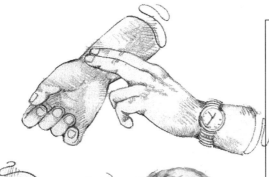

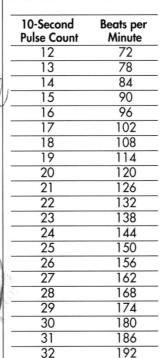

TABLE 2	
10-Second Pulse Count	Beats per Minute
12	72
13	78
14	84
15	90
16	96
17	102
18	108
19	114
20	120
21	126
22	132
23	138
24	144
25	150
26	156
27	162
28	168
29	174
30	180
31	186
32	192
33	198

sure your body is responding the way it should.

Measuring intensity.

How do you know when you are at 50% to 70% of your VO_2 max? You won't be able to measure your oxygen consumption during your normal workouts, but there are several good ways to tell how hard you're working. The most common way is to monitor your heart rate. As exercise becomes harder, your muscles need more oxygen and your heart must beat faster to deliver it. The direct relationship between heart rate and oxygen consumption allows you to measure exercise intensity simply by counting your pulse or by wearing an electronic heart rate monitor.

To count your pulse, place your first two fingers (not your thumb) over the radial artery, which is found in the top third of the inside of your other wrist on the thumb side, or over the carotid artery, which runs up the inside of your neck near the Adam's apple. Use light but firm pressure so that you can feel your pulse. You should feel a pulse each time your heart beats. Take a resting heart rate by counting the number of beats in 60 seconds while you are lying in bed before you get up in the morning.

To get an exercise heart rate, you will probably have to stop what you're doing briefly. Your heart slows down very quickly when you stop exercising, so be ready to count as soon as you can. Find your pulse while you

If you have complications of diabetes, your exercise intensity may have to be closely controlled to prevent you from running into problems. For example, if an exercise test shows that you get abnormal blood pressure or heart responses at a particular level of exercise, you may be told to keep your intensity well below the hazardous stage. This may be less than the recommended 50% to 70% VO_2 max. You should be given specific instructions on monitoring your workouts to make are still moving. Stop your exercise, but at least keep your legs moving by marching in place or continuing to walk. Count your pulse for 10 seconds and multiply by 6 to get the number of heart beats per minute (Table 2).

An alternative to counting your pulse is to purchase an electronic heart rate monitor. The most accurate monitors use electrodes worn on the chest that transmit a signal to a wristwatch or digital counter. Some models will store and record heart rate readings at set intervals throughout your workout, and others signal you if your heart rate is lower or higher than it should be. A high-quality, reliable monitor can be very helpful, but they are fairly expensive. Discuss this with your health-care team to see whether purchasing one would be a good idea for you.

How often should you check your heart rate?

You should always count your heart rate before you begin to exercise and after you have warmed up with 5 or 10 minutes of stretching and mild aerobic activity. You should check again after about 5 minutes of your aerobic workout to make sure you are at the right intensity. If your pulse is too high or too low, make adjustments by slowing down or speeding up and check again. You should also stop and check any time you feel any unusual symptoms such as dizziness, shortness of breath, nausea, changes in vision, or discomfort in your chest, neck, jaw, or arms. Count your pulse when you complete your aerobic workout and again after you have cooled down with 5 to 10 minutes of slower activity and more gentle stretching.

How fast should your heart rate be?

Ideally, you will be given a range of heart rates that have been found to be safe and effective for you during exercise testing and that represent an appropriate percentage of your VO_2 max. Often, people are given target heart rates for exercise based on general formulas using age as a basis for estimating maximal heart rates. A common one uses the formula 220 – age. However, approximations of maximal heart rate may be off by as much as 20 beats per minute or more in relatively healthy people without diabetes. If you take medications for your heart, blood pressure, or eyes that slow your heart rate, or if you have complications of diabetes that affect your heart rate response to exercise, such as autonomic neuropathy, an exercise test is the only way to be sure that a target heart rate is appropriate for your individual needs. It is far better to have an individualized prescription developed for your target heart rate than to rely on rough estimations.

Here's an example. Estimating target heart rates is usually done with the formula 220 – age (which estimates maximum heart rate). Subtract your resting heart rate from this number; this gives your heart rate reserve. Multiply your heart rate reserve by 0.5 or 0.7, then add your resting heart rate back to the result. This gives your target heart rate when working at 50% or 70% of your heart rate reserve (see Table 3, next page). A 33-year-old with a resting heart rate of 98 would have a heart rate reserve of 89 (220 – 33 = 187 – 98 = 89). This formula would give target heart rates of 143 at 50% of maximum capacity and 160 at 70% of maximum capacity (89 x 0.5 = 45 + 98 = 143; 89 x 0.7 = 62 + 98 = 160). But a 33 year old woman with type I diabetes had an exercise test and found that, due to autonomic neuropathy, her maximum heart rate was really 135, not 187. No matter how hard she exercises, her heart rate

How to Estimate Your Target Heart Rate

- To estimate your target heart rate for workouts, you first need to know your maximum heart rate and your resting heart rate.
- For maximum heart rate, use the rate determined during your exercise stress test, or use the estimation formula 220 – age. Note that an exercise stress test is the only way to be sure of your maximum heart rate. It is important to have an exercise stress test if you have autonomic neuropathy or take medications that can slow your heart rate.
- For resting heart rate, count your pulse for a full minute while you are relaxed and sitting down.
- Put these numbers into the formula:
  Maximum heart rate (HRmax) – resting heart rate (HRrest = heart rate maximum reserve (HRmax reserve)
- Multiply heart rate reserve by the lower and upper limits of work out intensity. The American Diabetes Association recommends you use the limits of 50% and 70%. Multiply heart rate reserve by 0.5 or 0.7.
- To find your target heart rates, add resting heart rate to the upper and lower percentages of heart rate reserve.

*To find a 10-second target heart rate, divide the target numbers by six. In example 2, during 10-second pulse checks, the man would aim for a 10-second pulse count of 20 if he is working at 50% of capacity or a 10-second pulse count of 24 if he is working at 70% of capacity.

Example 1:

A fifty-five-year-old woman with a resting heart rate of 84 and a maximum heart rate estimated by 220 – 55 = 165.

	Lower Limit	Upper Limit
HRmax	165	165
–HRrest	–84	–84
=HRmax reserve	81	81
x Intensity	x .50	x .70
= %HRmax reserve	41	57
+ HRrest	+ 84	+ 84
= Target HR	125	141

This tells the woman that she should aim for a heart rate of 125 beats per minute to work out at 50% of her heart's capacity or 141 beats per minute to work out at 70% of her heart's capacity.

Example 2:

A 38-year-old man with a resting heart rate of 72 and a maximum heart rate of 170 determined by exercise testing.

	Lower Limit	Upper Limit
HRmax	170	170
–HRrest	–72	–72
=HRmax reserve	98	98
x Intensity	x .50	x .70
= %HRmax reserve	49	69
+ HRrest	+ 72	+ 72
= Target HR*	121	141

This tells the man that he should aim for a heart rate of 121 beats per minute to work out at 50% of capacity or 141 beats per minute to work out at 70% of capacity.

will never rise above 135. To work at 50% to 70% of her maximal capacity, she needs to aim for a heart rate of 116 to 122 beats per minute.

With aerobic training, your resting pulse rate will become slower. Early into your new exercise program, count your heart rate. Count it for a full minute when you're relaxed and sitting or lying down. After several months of exercise, count your resting heart rate again. A lower resting heart rate will show that your heart is pumping more blood with less effort than when you were less fit. (Note that if you have autonomic neuropathy, you may not see this training effect on your heart rate.)

Another simple way to monitor exercise intensity is to rely on your own perceptions of how difficult the exercise feels. A scale known as the Rating of Perceived Exertion (RPE) compares very closely to more complicated monitoring methods such as percent of VO_2 max or heart rate. It may be especially useful if you have difficulty counting pulse rates or if you are on medications that slow your heart rate. The most common RPE scale uses numbers ranging from 6 to 20, with verbal descriptions of increasing fatigue at every odd number (Table 4).

Moderate aerobic exercise at 50% to 70% VO_2 max generally corresponds to RPE ratings of 11–14. You should be trained how to use the RPE method properly. Your ratings of exertion should match the more precise ways to monitor intensity. It is usually best to combine the RPE method with at least one additional technique, such as heart rate monitoring.

Exercise intensity can also be monitored by recording your pace or rate of performing physical work. You could write down how far and how fast you walk, swim, bicycle, or run. Scientists have very carefully measured

TABLE 4

RATING OF PERCEIVED EXERTION (RPE) SCALE

20
19 Very, Very Hard
18
17 Very Hard
16
15 Hard
14
13 Somewhat Hard
12
11 Fairly Light
10
9 Very Light
8
7 Very, Very Light
6

From Borg GA: *Med Sci Sports Exerc* 14: 377-387, 1982

how much oxygen is required to do most types of activity, so by knowing exactly what you do, it is fairly easy to calculate how much oxygen you are using. For example, if you were to tell an exercise physiologist that you walked one mile in 25 minutes, he or she would know that this exercise required 2.8 times more oxygen than you would use if you were just resting. This walking speed may be just what you need if the most oxygen you

TABLE 5
ENERGY COST OF EXERCISE

Activity	Pace or Type	METs	Activity	Pace or Type	METs
Walking	30 min/mile	2.5	Swimming	75 yards/min	11
Walking	24 min/mile	3	Running	8.5 min/mile	12
Dancing	Fox-trot, waltz	3	Bicycling	3.5 min/mile	12
Bicycling, stationary	50 watts	3	Rowing, stationary	200 watts	12
Walking	15 min/mile	4	Running	7 min/mile	14
Bicycling	6 min/mile	4	Cross-country skiing	<7.5 min/mile	14
Water aerobics	Beginner level	4	Running	6 min/mile	16
Aerobics	Beginner or low impact	5	Bicycling	<3 min/mile	16
Dancing	Folk, square	5.5			
Walk/Jog	14 min/mile	6			
Bicycling	5.5 min/mile	6			
Swimming	Leisurely	6			
Dancing	Ballet, modern	6			
Aerobics	Advanced or high impact	7			
Bicycling, stationary	150 watts	7			
Running	12 min/mile	8			
Bicycling	4.5 min/mile	8			
Swimming	50 yards/min	8			
Running	10 min/mile	10			
Bicycling	4 min/mile	10			

To convert METs to calories, use the formula:

[METs x body weight in pounds x minutes] ÷ 132 = calories

For example, if a 140-pound woman walked/jogged 2 miles in 28 minutes, she would have worked at 6 METs:

[6 x 140 x 28] ÷ 132 = 178 calories burned

From Ainsworth BE, et al.: Compendium of physical activities: classification of energy costs of human physical activities. *Med Sci Sports Exercise* 25:71-80, 1993

could consume during exercise was 5 or 6 times your resting level. If you tried to walk that mile in 12 minutes, you would be very close to your VO$_2$ max and would find it to be far too difficult. You could also record how much exercise you have done on a machine that measures exercise work loads in a unit of energy such as calories or other measurements of the rate of work such as watts or METs. Many fitness centers have ergometric bicycles, treadmills, stairclimbers, and rowing machines that measure the rate of work performed on them; this is often given as number of calories burned during a workout or watts being generated as you work out, for instance, on a rowing machine. Initial work loads can easily be set for individuals after an exercise test has been performed. As you become more aerobically fit, you will find that the same work loads or walking speeds have become easy and that you need to increase the work load. For this reason, it is best to monitor exercise intensity by work load or exercise pace in combination with heart rate or RPE monitoring.

More about METs.

As you learn more about exercise, you'll probably run into METs. Short for a unit of resting metabolism, a MET is a way to measure the intensity of exercise. Activities are assigned a particular MET depending on how much oxygen is consumed. For instance, at rest, you have an oxygen consumption considered to measure 1 MET. Walking at a pace of 1 mile every 30 minutes rates as 2.5 METs of work. If you increase your pace to 1 mile every 15 minutes, you are working at 4 METs. On average, this means that you are consuming 3.5 milliliters of oxygen per kilogram of body weight (1 kilogram = 2.2 pounds). If you are exercising at a rate that is four times your resting VO_2, you would be working at 4 METs.

If you know your workload in METs, you can estimate the number of calories you are using to exercise. If you work out on a machine that measures METs and also asks you how much you weigh, it can tell you approximately how many calories you are burning. If you are walking, running, biking, or swimming, see Table 5 to find the estimated METs for your workout. You will need to know the pace, such as how long it takes you to walk a mile or that it takes you 10 minutes to pedal a mile on your bike.

How Long Should I Exercise?

The recommended duration of aerobic exercise is 20 to 45 minutes, with additional time needed for warming up and cooling down. Your entire workout should take about one hour. Twenty minutes appears to be the minimal time needed to improve or maintain your VO_2 max, but this assumes you will work at a fairly high intensity. Most people prefer to reduce the intensity to a more comfortable level and lengthen the duration. Doing one type of exercise for more than 45 minutes, however, is associated with an unreasonably high rate of injuries, especially in activities that place great stress on the joints, such as running and stairclimbing.

Periods shorter than 20 minutes may be appropriate if you have certain exercise limitations. Several brief periods of exercise, spread throughout the day, may be needed if you are unable to exercise for the entire 20–45 minutes in one session. Much shorter periods of exercise can also be used when you're first starting out, especially if you have been inactive for many years. It's far better to start out exercising for 2 minutes on your first day and take 2 years to reach an exercise program lasting 30 minutes than to start out exercising for 45 minutes and stop the next day.

How Often Should I Exercise?

Most people should exercise 3 to 5 days per week. Little or no improvements in fitness will be seen with only 1 or 2 exercise periods per week, and injuries become all too common with more than 5 weekly workout sessions. Your body requires some rest time. The improvements in insulin sensitivity that occur because of exercise last, at most, only 2 or 3 days, so try to space your workouts as evenly as possible throughout the

MY EXERCISE PLAN

Name: _____ Date:_____

Physician: _____ Phone: _____

Exercise physiologist: _____ Phone: _____

Type of activity: _____ Frequency: _____ Duration: _____

Intensity to be monitored by:_____ Heart rate: _____

Distance/time: _____

Work load: _____

RPE: _____

Best times for exercise: _____

_____

Blood glucose monitoring schedule: _____

_____

_____

_____

Adjustments for exercise:
Food or drink: _____

_____

_____

_____

Insulin: _____

_____

_____

_____

Special precautions: _____

_____

_____

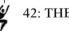

week. When weight loss is the primary goal, 5 exercise sessions per week will get you the best results.

WHERE DO I START?

Think of exercise as a project for a lifetime. Start slowly and build gradually. You should develop an exercise plan designed to meet the goals you have set. Your plan should include the type of activity you will do, along with the intensity and how it should be monitored, plus the frequency, and duration (Table 6). Your health-care team should recommend the best time of day for you to exercise. If you take insulin or oral hypoglycemic medications, you need a specific plan for monitoring your blood glucose. Your plan should also include adjustments in diet or insulin therapy to anticipate changes in blood glucose. If hypoglycemia develops, you should know what food, drink, or glucose upplements should be taken to get you back on track, and what to do to prevent any further drops in your blood glucose level into the hypoglycemic range.

Talk to your health-care team about organized exercise programs in your area. If you have long-term complications, consider at least beginning your exercise program under medical supervision. Many health-care delivery systems, hospitals, and universities have exercise physiologists and other expert staff that can help you get off on the right foot. They should be able to help you find just the right intensity level and can work closely with you to make sure you are exercising safely.

KEEPING AN EXERCISE LOG

Record keeping is an indispensable part of your exercise plan. An exercise log book will help you focus on your goals and will enable you to track your accomplishments. Record keeping will help you learn how your body reacts, so you can figure out what works and what doesn't work for you. Your log book can provide important information to your doctor and other members of your health-care team to indicate what adjustments to make to your medication and eating plan. Together you should be able to make any necessary changes so that you can get the most out of exercise while minimizing problems. Consider using one of the sample logs found in Tables 7–9 or use this information to create your personal exercise log. ❧

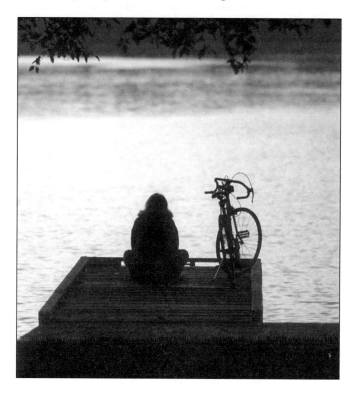

TABLE 7

EXERCISE LOG FOR PEOPLE WITH TYPE I DIABETES

Date: _____   Time of day: _____

Weather conditions: _____   Where exercise was done: _____

BEFORE

Blood glucose: _____   Time taken: _____

Urine checked for ketones (if glucose is >250 mg/dl) ☐ Positive   ☐ Negative

Heart rate: _____   Blood pressure: _____

Food or drink: _____   Time of day: _____

Insulin: Type: _____Dosage:_____   Injection site: _____

DURING

Warm-up activity: _____   Duration: _____

Heart rate after warm up: _____   Blood pressure after warm up: _____

Exercise activity: _____   Duration: _____

Intensity: _____   Heart rate: _____

Blood pressure: _____   Distance/time:_____

Work load: _____   RPE: _____

Blood glucose: _____   Time taken: _____

Food or drink: _____   Time of day: _____

AFTER

Cool-down activity: _____   Duration: _____

Heart rate after cool down: _____   Blood pressure after cool down: _____

Blood glucose: _____   Time taken: _____

Food or drink: _____   Time of day: _____

Feet checked for irritations, blisters: ☐ Yes ☐ No

Additional blood glucose test: _____   Time taken: _____

Additional blood glucose test: _____   Time taken: _____

Comments: _____
_____
_____

Note that you may not need to collect all of this information each time you exercise. However, having this information will help you and your health-care team spot and solve problems.

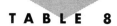

EXERCISE LOG FOR PEOPLE WITH TYPE II DIABETES WHO TAKE INSULIN OR ORAL HYPOGLYCEMIC AGENTS

Date: _____ Time of day: _____

Weather conditions: _____ Where exercise was done: _____

BEFORE

Blood glucose: _____ Time taken: _____

Urine checked for ketones (if glucose is >250 mg/dl) ☐ Positive   ☐ Negative

Heart rate: _____ Blood pressure: _____

Food or drink: _____ Time of day: _____

Insulin: Type: _____ Dosage: _____ Injection site: _____

Oral Agent: Type: _____ Dosage: _____ Time taken: _____

DURING

Warm-up activity: _____ Duration: _____

Heart rate after warm up: _____ Blood pressure after warm up: _____

Exercise activity: _____ Duration: _____

Intensity: _____ Heart rate: _____

Blood pressure: _____ Distance/time: _____

Work load: _____ RPE: _____

Blood glucose: _____ Time taken: _____

Food or drink: _____ Time of day: _____

AFTER

Cool-down activity: _____ Duration: _____

Heart rate after cool down: _____ Blood pressure after cool down: _____

Blood glucose: _____ Time taken: _____

Food or drink: _____ Time of day: _____

Feet checked for irritations, blisters: ☐ Yes ☐ No

Additional blood glucose test: _____ Time taken: _____

Additional blood glucose test: _____ Time taken: _____

Comments: _____

Note that you may not need to collect all of this information each time you exercise. However, having this information will help you and your health-care team spot and solve problems.

TABLE 9

EXERCISE LOG FOR PEOPLE WITH TYPE II DIABETES TREATED BY DIET AND EXERCISE

Date: _____   Time of day: _____

Weather conditions: _____   Where exercise was done: _____

BEFORE

Blood glucose: _____   Time taken: _____

Heart rate before exercise: _____   Blood pressure before exercise: _____

DURING

Warm-up activity: _____   Duration: _____

Heart rate after warm up: _____   Blood pressure after warm up: _____

Exercise activity: _____   Duration: _____

Intensity: _____   Heart rate: _____

Blood pressure: _____   Distance/time:_____

Work load: _____   RPE: _____

Blood glucose: _____   Time taken: _____

Food or drink: _____   Time of day: _____

AFTER

Cool-down activity: _____   Duration: _____

Heart rate after cool down: _____   Blood pressure after cool down: _____

Blood glucose: _____   Time taken: _____

Feet checked for irritations, blisters: ☐ Yes ☐ No

Comments: _____

_____

_____

_____

_____

Note that you may not need to collect all of this information each time you exercise. However, having this information will help you and your health-care team spot and solve problems.

CHAPTER 5

Security is mostly a
superstition. It does not exist
in nature, nor do the
children of men as a whole
experience it. Avoiding
danger is no safer in the long
run than outright exposure.
Life is either a daring
adventure, or nothing.

—Helen Keller

Exercising
Safely

YOU'VE MADE IT OVER THE FIRST HURDLE
AND SELECTED THE BEST EXERCISE
PROGRAM FOR YOU. Along with your health-
care team, you have made an honest and careful
assessment of your health status and decided
what exercises will be right for you. Now that you're ready to
begin an exercise program, the biggest challenge lies ahead—
avoiding the problems that will make you stop excerising.

Don't trip yourself up just as you get started by trying to
do too much too soon. Exercising too long or too hard at first
increases your chances for injury. The other consideration is

blood glucose control. Your blood glucose level will respond to exercise, but everyone with diabetes is different. If you take insulin or oral glucose-lowering medications, take time to become familiar with this response and to gradually increase the intensity and duration of exercise so you can minimize your chances of developing hypoglycemia. Nothing can shake your confidence like unexpected hypoglycemia.

Learning how to keep your blood glucose level in balance during exercise means that you will need to do things you may not have done before. Most people with diabetes who exercise succeed through trial and error. Try not to let this challenge keep you from attempting new things. To adapt to regular exercise, you'll probably need to make changes in your diabetes care regimen. You may need less insulin or oral hypoglycemic medication or more food. Self-monitoring your blood glucose levels minimizes your risks by allowing you to understand your response to exercise and make adjustments.

Don't be discouraged if, after beginning an exercise program, your glucose control is temporarily less than ideal. This happens to almost everyone. Don't be discouraged if you have more episodes of hypoglycemia than usual. These are problems that you can solve by learning new behaviors, like blood testing before and after exercising and adjusting your medication dosage.

EXERCISE AND BLOOD GLUCOSE LEVELS

Starting to exercise when you've been away from it for awhile is like being dealt a new hand of cards in a card game. The players are the same, but you're playing with a slightly different set of numbers, so you need to adjust your strategy. Luckily, we know some things about how exercise reshuffles the metabolism. For instance, exercise increases the effectiveness of naturally produced or injected insulin. This means that the same amount of insulin may lower blood glucose levels more than expected. Exercise also increases the rate at which the muscles take up glucose and other energy-providing nutrients. This means that insulin may start to work faster than normal. On the other hand, high-intensity exercise can promote glucose release from the liver into the blood. This means that sometimes exercise can increase blood glucose levels. Because of these factors, you'll need to be on the lookout for hypoglycemia and hyperglycemia.

GOING LOW

Hypoglycemia due to exercise may occur in people with type I diabetes or people with type II diabetes who are treated with insulin or oral glucose-lowering medications. People who control type II diabetes with diet and exercise generally do not encounter exercise-related hypoglycemia.

Hypoglycemia can occur during or after exercise as the glucose that was used to fuel the exercise is returned to the muscles and as the action of insulin is enhanced by exercise. Eating can help control this exercise-created low blood glucose. But, there are factors that you can't control that affect the ability of insulin to lower your glucose level. Despite your attempts to be consistent, injecting the same amount of insulin can have results that vary from day to day, by as much as 25 percent. Adding the effects of exercise (increased blood flow and body temperature) to this normal variation in insulin action can lead to hypoglycemia even if you don't change anything else. So, although you think you've covered your bases, you can go low because of exercise. This is why testing is your best defense against hypoglycemia. See Table 1 for some strategies that may help you avoid hypoglycemia.

Delayed hypoglycemia.

When you exercise, the energy comes from glucose that muscles and the liver make from their stores of glycogen. If you exercise hard or for a long time, your glycogen stores will run very low. As this source of glucose runs out, some glucose is taken from the blood to fuel the activity. This can cause blood glucose levels to drop somewhat while you work out. However, blood glucose levels can also drop after you've finished exercising. This is because your body rebuilds its supply of glycogen in the muscles and liver by taking glucose from the blood until the stores are full once again. So, for hours, sometimes up to and beyond 24 hours, your body needs the glucose you get from meals to resupply your glycogen stores. This is how exercise can cause hypoglycemia long after the exercise is over. Postexercise hypoglycemia is much more common than hypoglycemia during exercise.

GOING HIGH

You're about to start an aerobics class, so you test your blood glucose. Your blood glucose is about 200 mg/dl. From previous experience, you know that the exercise will bring your glucose level down, yet you won't have to worry about going too low, if you stick to

---

TABLE 1

STRATEGIES FOR AVOIDING HYPOGLYCEMIA

- Exercise 1 to 3 hours after you eat.
- Learn your individual glucose response to different types of exercise by monitoring your blood glucose before, during, and after exercising.
- Test your blood glucose twice before you exercise, 30 minutes apart, to know whether your blood glucose level is stable or dropping.
- Avoid exercising when your insulin is peaking; be aware that exercise increases blood flow, which increases how fast your insulin goes to work.
- Decrease the insulin dose that will be working while you exercise.
- You may need to eat during or after exercise if you exercise vigorously or for a long time (an hour or more).
- Be aware that you may need extra food for up to 24 hours after exercising, depending on how hard and how long you exercised.

Adapted from Horton ES: *Exercise.* In *Therapy for Diabetes* Mellitus *and Related Disorders.* Lebovitz HE, Ed. Alexandria, VA, Am. Diabetes Assoc., 1990, p. 110

---

working out at your usual intensity and duration.

Your health-care team has probably told you that exercise is a positive way to bring down blood glucose levels. But where exercise and blood glucose levels are concerned, the saying, "if a little is good, more is better," does not apply. If your fasting blood glucose level is greater than 300 mg/dl, whether you have type I or type II diabetes, your diabetes is in poor control and you need to check with your doctor to make sure it's okay for you to exercise.

If you have type I diabetes and your preexercise glucose test is over 250 mg/dl, stop and test your urine ketones. If you test negative for ketones, you can

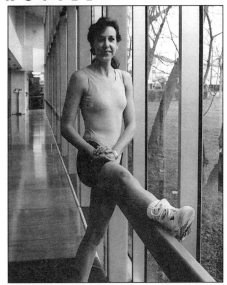

"I AM MORE IN CONTROL OF THIS DISEASE THAN IT IS OF ME."

Exercise is second nature to fitness professional Chris Silkwood. She grew up playing softball and enjoying sports. When she was diagnosed with type I diabetes 12 years ago, she says "exercise was my saving grace."

Now director of the Diabetes Treatment Center at Park Plaza Hospital in Houston, Texas, and president of Silkwood Enterprises, a Houston-based fitness services firm, Chris remembers how different things were when she was diagnosed.

"It took me a long time to understand good diabetes management because resources weren't available when I was first diagnosed. My physician mailed me the Exchange Lists and said, 'Here you go.' By no means was it the most positive way to start. I had to do a lot of self education—reading materials, talking to health-care professionals." Memories of her own struggle to become informed help fuel her commitment and enthusiasm for her work in diabetes education today.

Chris credits exercise with helping her cope from the beginning. Chris says not only has regular exercise helped her control her blood glucose levels and kept her cardiovascular system strong, but it's also given her a new perspective on living with diabetes. "Exercise healed me in terms of attitude and feeling that I had a sense of control over my body even though it was being attacked by this disease. Exercise helps me feel that I am more in control of this disease than it is of me."

Chris believes that a regular program of exercise can help you cope with whatever life dishes out. Being alive means facing crisis and stress. But Chris says, "I'm a true believer that if you are taking care of your body, those crises don't become the kind of thing that consume you. Crises will come along, but if you are taking care of yourself, there's a greater likelihood that you can take care of the crisis."

Both professionally and personally, Chris practices what she preaches. An advocate of cross-training, she enjoys a variety of aerobic activities including running, cycling, teaching aerobics classes, stairclimbing, and weight training. Chris not only teaches aerobics but has a local television exercise show. Recently, Chris added boxing lessons to her repertoire. Boxing attracted her because it was so different and something that she could do just for herself. Boxing gives her a new fitness challenge in an environment where no one calls on her for instruction. In fact, at the boxing gym, she has had to struggle with learning completely new skills. "Sports were always very easy, and this was something totally new. It was a real challenge. It was exciting for me to get into something that I wasn't good at and to see my skill level improve."

While boxing may only bring to mind images of professionals slugging it out in the ring, Chris jokes that she has no interest in hitting someone. What she was interested in was a fresh physical challenge. Workouts at the gym provide this. "Boxing is great for developing upper body strength and for stress management," she says.

What about working out in such a traditionally male sport? "There was a little intimidation in the beginning," admits Chris. But she's quick to add that when you work hard, you earn the respect of others.

Chris encourages her students to

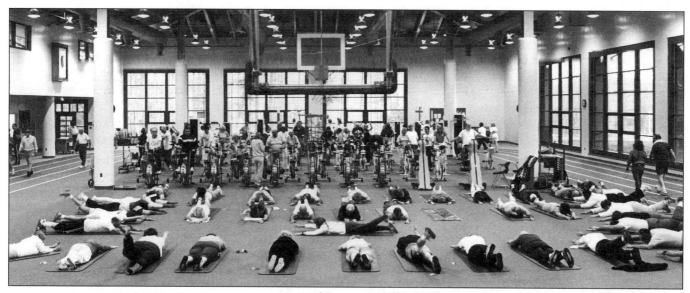

Don't forget to stretch. Photograph by Les Todd, courtesy of Duke University Photo Department.

experiment and challenge themselves with new forms of exercise. "Generally I encourage people to take a shopping spree with exercise and try a variety of different kinds of activity to see what suits them best." To find an exercise you'll stick with, Chris advises doing something you enjoy and something at which you feel proficient. If you feel awkward and uncomfortable, chances are you won't stick with it.

Chris works out daily and tests her blood glucose three times a day: a fasting morning level, a preexercise level, and before-bed level. She finds that an occasional high blood glucose level is inevitable, but generally she maintains good control. Her prescription for avoiding exercise-induced reactions? Do not ignore low blood glucose levels. "I think it's very important for people with diabetes, whether they exercise or not, to drop any kind of heroic attitude toward ignoring low blood glucose levels. They need to overcome any sense of embarrassment and learn to speak up about low blood glucose. They need to be able to do what is necessary to treat themselves or ask for help."

As a member of the President's Council on Physical Fitness and Sports (see Resources), Chris has been able to work for children's fitness. "Illinois is the only state where physical education is mandatory at the elementary level," she says. "In Texas, the average child gets less than 20 minutes per week of physical education. That's outrageous." Through her work with the American Diabetes Association camp program in Texas, Chris helps get the fitness message out to children with diabetes.

Diabetes education has come a long way in the 12 years since Chris' diagnosis. Chris Silkwood, both through her work and her example, helps people with diabetes toward a better quality of life. ■

exercise but be sure to monitor your blood glucose level during and after exercise. If you test positive for ketones, you may not have enough insulin in your body. In this situation, if you go ahead and exercise, you could drive blood glucose levels even higher. Why?

Glucose levels can increase during exercise if they are already high for this reason: high-intensity exercise (defined as what's high intensity for *your* body, which could be walking a mile faster than usual or pedaling your bike up a steep hill) can stimulate your liver to break down stores of glycogen to create glucose. You might discover by testing that your postexercise blood glucose level is even higher than when you started. If you have enough insulin available, your blood glucose will recover rapidly. But if your levels of insulin are low, you could start producing ketones. Although exercise-induced hyperglycemia can occur in both type I and type II diabetes, problems with ketones only happen in type I diabetes.

Ketosis.

Ketones are produced in the liver as a by-product of fat breakdown. When your body needs fuel and not enough glucose is available (even though glucose levels may be high) because the insulin "key" hasn't unlocked the "gate" to let glucose into the muscles and other tissues, fat will be used for fuel instead. This happens when too little insulin is available, which is why it is primarily a problem for people with type I diabetes.

Ketones are acid substances. When amounts are high, ketones disrupt your body's chemical balance. In essence, too many ketones in the blood, called ketosis, will dehydrate the body's cells. Your body can handle small amounts of ketones; they are a normal waste

product of your body's life-sustaining processes and are disposed of in the urine. However, when too many ketones are produced, the chemical imbalance can overwhelm the body. This process, called ketoacidosis, usually takes several hours to occur. But if insulin levels remain low, ketoacidosis is a health risk that, if not properly treated and monitored, can result in coma and death. Ketoacidosis can occur in people with undiagnosed type I diabetes.

If you require insulin injections to control diabetes, whether you have type I or type II diabetes, you are at risk for exercise-induced hyperglycemia if you start exercising when your blood glucose level is over 250 mg/dl and, for people with type I diabetes, if a urine test reveals moderate or large amounts of ketones. You could risk worsening the ketosis. (See How to Self-Test, pages 54 and 55.) Your insulin levels are too low. Don't exercise until your urine ketone levels test at trace or negative amounts. Confirm that your doctor agrees with your use of these guidelines.

YOU DON'T SELF-MONITOR? READ THIS

It's tough to underestimate the benefits of self-monitoring blood glucose. Self-monitoring blood glucose is your primary key to learning about how your body reacts to exercise (and food and stress and airline travel and on and on). It is the cornerstone of safe exercise. It is your passport to a more flexible lifestyle and, in essence, freedom.

Testing before and after exercise is the safest thing to do. For most people, a safe preexercise blood glucose level is between 100 and 250 mg/dl (Table 2).

■ If you try a new activity, or work out longer or harder than usual, do a blood test.

TABLE 2

PREVENTING AN INSULIN REACTION

- Plan ahead
- Test your blood glucose before you start exercising
  - If under 100 mg/dl, eat a snack, then test again in 20 to 30 minutes
  - If 100 to 150 mg/dl, exercise, but test during and after exercise and eat a snack afterward, if necessary
  - If 151 to 250 mg/dl, okay to exercise
  - If over 250 but less than 300 mg/dl and you have type II diabetes, okay to exercise*
  - If over 250 but less that 300 mg/dl and you have type I diabetes, test urine for ketones
    - If ketones are moderate or high, you don't have enough insulin; wait to exercise until ketone testing shows negative or trace amounts
    - If ketones are negative, okay to exercise*

*If fasting blood glucose is over 300 mg/dl and you have type I or type II diabetes, you probably should not exercise until you are in better control—you need to check with your doctor first

- Carry a fast-acting carbohydrate to use if you become hypoglycemic, such as
  - Regular soft drink
  - Glucose tablets
  - Glucose gels
  - Raisins

- Do a blood test after every 30 minutes of continuous exercise.
- If you feel the symptoms of an insulin reaction, stop and test.

See the section on How to Self-Test.

You can double the reward of testing by remembering to write down your test results. Not only do you learn what's going on at the time you do the test, but you can see patterns in your blood glucose levels over time when you review your results. Write your results in a log book so that you can learn about your body.

Remember that the effects of exercise that cause your blood glucose level to drop occur most often after you exercise. Therefore, on days that you exercise,

- Test your blood before meals and before going to bed (if you don't already).
- If you are low, eat a snack before going to sleep: You want to avoid hypoglycemia while you sleep.
- If you've exercised longer or harder than usual or changed your exercise routine, remember that your tests in the next 2 to 24 hours could reflect this exertion.

If you've had recurring problems with hypoglycemia during the night, plan on eating before going to sleep and testing your blood about midway through your sleep (around 2 or 3 A.M.). If the results show that your blood glucose levels have dropped since your bedtime test, make sure you eat before going back to sleep. You should test frequently if you feel the symptoms of an insulin reaction or have trouble recognizing these symptoms.

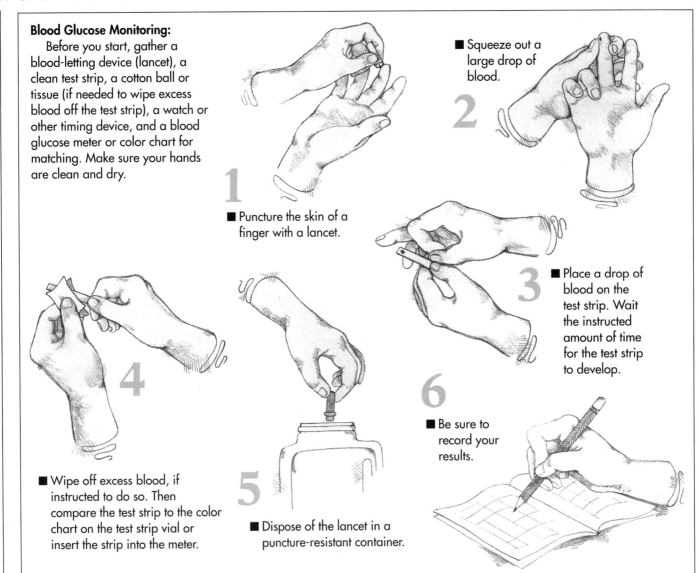

Blood Glucose Monitoring:

Before you start, gather a blood-letting device (lancet), a clean test strip, a cotton ball or tissue (if needed to wipe excess blood off the test strip), a watch or other timing device, and a blood glucose meter or color chart for matching. Make sure your hands are clean and dry.

1 ■ Puncture the skin of a finger with a lancet.

2 ■ Squeeze out a large drop of blood.

3 ■ Place a drop of blood on the test strip. Wait the instructed amount of time for the test strip to develop.

4 ■ Wipe off excess blood, if instructed to do so. Then compare the test strip to the color chart on the test strip vial or insert the strip into the meter.

5 ■ Dispose of the lancet in a puncture-resistant container.

6 ■ Be sure to record your results.

Urine Ketone Monitoring:

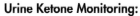

Before you start, gather a clean test strip, a cup for collecting urine (unless you put test strip into the urine stream), a watch or other timing device, and color chart for matching.

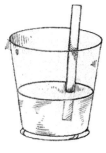

1

■ Dip test strip in collected urine or pass it through the urine stream.

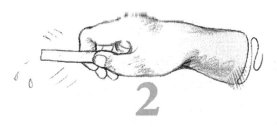

2

■ Gently shake the test strip to remove excess urine.

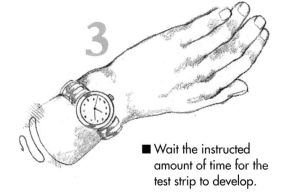

3

■ Wait the instructed amount of time for the test strip to develop.

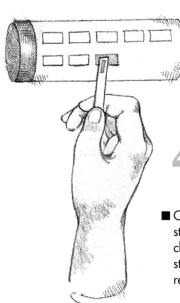

4

■ Compare the test strip to the color chart on the test strip vial. Be sure to record your results.

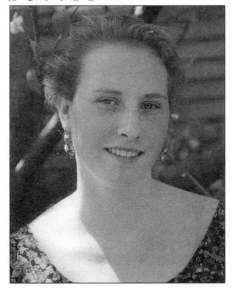

"I JUST TELL MYSELF, YOU CAN
DO IT." Competitive swimmers. We're
probably most aware of these athletes
during the Olympic Summer Games. We
watch spellbound as their streamlined
bodies churn up lap lanes with machine-
like precision. Years and years of training
all come down to this: Going for the Gold.
Back at home, thousands of young
swimmers put in their pool time. Lap after
lap. And they dream of making it to Junior
Nationals and then, Nationals, or of
nailing down a college scholarship. And
somewhere tucked in the back of their
minds is the ultimate dream: the Olympics.

Caroline Bridges is a 15-year-old
competitive swimmer in Atlanta, Georgia.

A glimpse at her workout schedule shows
just how dedicated young swimmers must
be. Bridges, a student at Pace Academy,
swims for the Swim Atlanta team. For
now, she favors the 50-yard freestyle but
competes in several different events at
meets.

During the school year Caroline swims
from 4:30 to 6:30 P.M. Monday through
Friday. On Saturdays she competes in a
meet or trains from 8 to 10 A.M. Swim
team members supplement these
workouts with weight training. Caroline
also swims and trains during the summer
months as well.

Caroline has had type I diabetes since
she was four. She has loved swimming
just as long. She's determined not to let
diabetes stand in her way. By planning
ahead, she works to avert potential
problems. For example, she
always has juice in her swim
bag. "If my blood glucose gets
low during practice, I get out of
the pool and get some," she
says.

Working out with
teammates helps improve
everyone's swimming, says
Caroline. "We really push
each other in practice."

Does she get prerace jitters?
"I get really nervous, but I just
tell myself, you can do it."
Sometimes premeet anxiety
can raise her blood glucose

level, and Caroline has to adjust her
insulin dosage accordingly.

Swim team members frequently travel
to out-of-town meets, something that
tends to raise her mother's anxiety level.
But while mom Susan Bridges may fret
about an unexpected occurrence, she
believes that recognizing and taking care
of low blood glucose reactions is
something that her daughter will have to
do on her own and that it's an issue of
being in control not only of her diabetes
but also of her own life.

Caroline may compete in eight or nine
meets during the school season and seven
meets in the summer. For the moment, she
seems focused on her short-term goal: To
reach Junior Nationals. Beyond that? A
scholarship to a college with a good swim
program would be just fine with her. ■

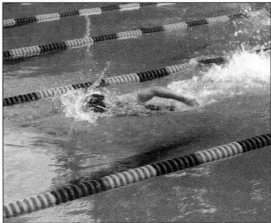

Caroline churns down a lane.

How Blood Glucose Levels Respond to Exercise

Several things influence how your blood glucose level responds to exercise. These include the type of exercise you choose, the intensity with which you exercise, and the length of time you spend exercising. For example, if you exercise long and hard, you are probably going to deplete glycogen stores in the muscles and liver that will be replaced by taking glucose from your blood.

When and what you ate at your most recent meal and your level of fitness also influence what happens to your blood glucose level while you exercise. If your most recent meal was more than three hours ago, you'll probably need to eat again so that your body has enough glucose to fuel the exercise. If the insulin you injected has its peak activity while you're exercising (a situation you want to avoid), even more glucose will be removed from your blood by the insulin.

The type of insulin you inject and the dosage and schedule you're on can affect your diabetes management while you exercise. You will need to do some trial and error experimenting to find your ideal balance between insulin and glucose.

Tailoring Your Glucose Control Plan

No one set of rules on blood glucose works for all people. The responses of blood glucose levels during and after exercise vary from person to person. Because each of us is unique in the way our body responds to exercise, we, together with our health-care team, need to design our own program for adjusting insulin, oral glucose-lowering medication, and diet for exercise.

Generally, you should exercise 1 to 3 hours after eating a meal. If you don't exercise after a meal or if you are practicing very tight blood glucose control, consider eating extra carbohydrate (10 to 15 grams of carbohydrate for every 30 minutes of planned exercise) before you start (see Table 3 for examples) or during your workout. For example, a college basketball player might drink eight ounces of a nondiet soda for every hour of practice. An alternative to eating is to have less insulin active in your body during your exercise session. This means decreasing the amount of insulin that will be working during the time you are exercising. You need to work out some experimental plans with your health-care team.

You'll find you need to make the most changes when you begin a new exercise program. When the changes work, most people stick with them. For instance, one young girl spends almost every day during the summer swimming and playing at the pool. For the summer, her mother cuts her insulin dose in half. Most changes aren't nearly that big. A serious cyclist reduces his Regular lunch insulin by 2 units on the days he takes his prelunch four-hour rides. He washes away his thirst with eight ounces of ginger ale (about 28 grams of carbohydrate) every hour during his ride.

You and your health-care team might decide to modify your insulin dose to accommodate your exercise plan. For instance, they may suggest that you try reducing your insulin dose that will be active during exercise by 20 to 40 percent of your usual dose. The serious cyclist has found that he has been able to cut his total daily insulin dose by about 25 percent since he started his workout program. His dose goes back up, however, if he misses his usual routine because of illness or an injury.

To help you and your doctor determine what adjustments to make, you need to write down pertinent

TABLE 3

CARBOHYDRATE REPLACEMENT

- The best way to determine whether you need extra food for exercise is to monitor your blood glucose levels before, during, and after exercise.
- In general, you should eat 10 to 15 grams of carbohydrate during or after exercising to replace that lost during every 30 minutes of vigorous exercise or every hour of moderate exercise. Examples are

  ¾ cup Cheerios
  ½ bagel
  3 cups plain popcorn
  1 small apple or peach
  12 cherries
  7 dried apricot halves
  ½ cup low-fat ice cream
  6 vanilla wafers
  4 ounces of a regular (nondiet) soft drink
  sports drink: consult label for amount

- Replace carbohydrate within two hours after exercising to reduce your risk of postexercise hypoglycemia.
- Remember to drink plenty of water.

- Record your blood glucose level readings before and after exercising.
- Keep a record of the time, intensity, and duration of the exercise you do and food or drink you take during exercise.

Like anyone who starts an exercise program, you'll want to begin gradually—exercising for short periods at first and gradually building up the amount of time and intensity at which you exercise. This will give you the chance to make changes in food or medication a little at a time.

A lot of people find that they have better diabetes control when they exercise at the same time every day. They've learned from their regular routine how much to eat and how soon after eating they can start to exercise. And they learn when to inject their insulin and how much they need. If you're having trouble controlling your diabetes during exercise, try to exercise at the same time each day.

INSULIN ACTION DURING EXERCISE

People who take insulin generally want to avoid exercising when their insulin peaks (Table 4). When this is impossible, test your blood glucose twice before you exercise, 30 minutes apart. This will tell you whether your blood glucose level is stable or dropping. If both insulin and exercise are taking glucose from your blood, this could result in hypoglycemia unless you eat extra carbohydrate.

Because exercise increases blood flow, exercising right after your injection can speed the action of insulin unpredictably. An injection site above an exercising

information. You may want to include this information in your exercise log (see Chapter 4). Keeping an exercise log helps you track your progress toward your goal.

- Keep a record of your insulin dose and the food you eat before you exercise.
- If you take oral medications (hypoglycemic agents and other medicines), keep a record of when you take them.

muscle will absorb insulin quicker than usual, taking up glucose from the blood faster than usual, leading to hypoglycemia. So, a good rule of thumb is to wait at least an hour after injecting insulin to begin to exercise. If this is not possible, you should at least try to inject insulin at a site that won't be used much during your workout. If you are tempted to interrupt your injection rotation routine because of exercise, you need to know that injecting into a site you don't normally use will cause some variation in insulin delivery. The abdominal injection site gives the most consistent absorption of insulin and provides the least variation in release of insulin. If you exercise frequently, you may want to talk with your health-care team about using the abdomen for all injections. You'll need to be sure to consistently rotate injection sites within the abdomen.

TABLE 4

GENERAL INSULIN ACTION TIMES

Insulin Type	Onset (hours)	Peak (hours)	Usual Effective Duration (hours)	Usual Maximum Duration (hours)
Animal				
Regular	0.5–2.0	3–4	4–6	6–8
NPH	4–6	8–14	16–20	20–24
Lente	4–6	8–14	16–20	20–24
Ultralente	8–14	Minimal	24–36	24–36
Human				
Regular	0.5–1.0	2–3	3–6	4–6
NPH	2–4	4–10	10–16	14–18
Lente	3–4	4–12	12–18	16–20
Ultralente	6–10	?	18–20	20–30

LISTENING TO YOUR BODY

As you exercise, pay attention to your body's warning signs. If you feel pain, other than the mild discomfort of working out, stop. The adage "no pain, no gain," has been changed to "feel pain, no gain." When you feel pain, your body is trying to tell you something usually that you're overdoing it and could be on the road to injury.

In addition, you'll need to watch for your symptoms of hypoglycemia. If you've had diabetes for a while, you know the symptoms, including shakiness or dizziness, faintness, blurred vision, irritability, clumsy or jerky movements, headache, moodiness, inattention or confusion, and hunger. Recognizing the symptoms of hypoglycemia can be more difficult during exercise because some of the symptoms—such as increased pulse rate and sweating—are also the signs of a healthy workout.

Learning to recognize hypoglycemia while exercising may take some practice. Some people have difficulty doing this, and almost everyone misses detecting the symptoms sometimes. If you consistently fail to recognize the symptoms, you'll need to test your blood glucose frequently during your exercise routine.

Treating hypoglycemia: for insulin users.

Whenever you feel the symptoms of hypoglycemia, stop and test your blood. If you are low, eat or drink 10 to 15 grams of fast-acting carbohydrate, such as four ounces of juice, half of a regular (nondiet) soft drink, glucose tablets or glucose gel, or pieces of hard candy— whatever you've found works best. Follow it up with a snack if your next meal isn't going to be within an hour. Don't forget that sometimes a rapid decrease in blood glucose level, even though it is still within target ranges, can feel like a hypoglycemic reaction.

After a hypoglycemic reaction, you can exercise again once your blood glucose level has returned to within your target range and the symptoms of the insulin reaction have disappeared—but not before.

Treating hypoglycemia: for oral medication users.

If you take oral glucose-lowering medications for type II diabetes, exercise can enhance the glucose-lowering effect and cause low blood glucose, much as it would in someone who takes insulin. These diabetes medications work to prompt your pancreas to produce more insulin. If you produce too much natural insulin while at the same time lowering your blood glucose level with exercise, your blood glucose level could drop too low.

Until you are used to your exercise routine and are familiar with the response exercise has on your diabetes control, test your blood glucose level before and after you exercise. If your blood glucose level goes too low, you need to treat the reaction. Take 10 to 15 grams of a fast-acting carbohydrate, such as four ounces of juice, half a regular (nondiet) soda, glucose tablets or gels, or pieces of hard candy. Follow it up with a snack if your next meal isn't going to be within an hour. You do not need to eat extra food before you exercise to avoid hypoglycemia like some people who inject insulin.

For you, even one episode of hypoglycemia during exercise means that you probably need to adjust your medication dose or diet. Talk to your doctor. Exercise can make your body more efficient in using the insulin it produces—cells are more receptive to the insulin and open up to let more glucose in. This is an increase in insulin sensitivity. If exercise is successful in increasing your body's sensitivity to insulin and lowering your weight, your doctor might cut down on your oral medication dosage or perhaps eliminate it completely.

DIET-MANAGED DIABETES AND BLOOD GLUCOSE

Those of you who have type II diabetes and manage it solely with diet don't need to regularly monitor your blood glucose or make changes in your food intake to exercise safely. Your body typically adjusts to the exercise much like someone who doesn't have diabetes. However, self-monitoring before and after exercise can help motivate you to stick with your exercise routine. It will show you how effective exercise is in lowering your blood glucose level.

Regular exercise will, over time, help your body become better at using the insulin it produces. You have type II diabetes because your body is not properly using the insulin it produces or it is not producing enough insulin to meet its needs.

Insulin plays the important role of allowing glucose to enter the cells in your body so it can be used for energy. Exercise can help make your body more receptive to insulin. As your tissues become more sensitive to the insulin your body makes, more glucose can move into the cells, thus reducing the amount of glucose left circulating in the blood. You want to avoid high blood glucose levels, because over time elevated blood glucose levels can lead to diabetes complications such as eye, heart, or kidney disease.

AVOIDING EXERCISE INJURY

There are two great ways to minimize your risk of exercise injury. One is to warm up and then stretch before you start exercising and then cool down and stretch afterward. The other is to gradually build up your exercise intensity and duration over many weeks or months. Your body will let you know when you've overdone it. Pain in the days following a workout is the signal that you've done too much. Often, exercise injuries to elbows and knees occur because they haven't had time to rest between exercise sessions.

The idea behind warming up is to get your muscles and heart ready for the demands of exercise. It's best to warm up for 5 to 10 minutes before the aerobic portion of your exercise routine begins. Your warm-up can include some low-intensity exercises such as walking or light calisthenics. Once your body is warm and feels "loose," include some stretching. Do not stretch before your warm-up. Stretching helps keep muscles flexible. When muscles and joints are tight and inflexible, they are more susceptible to injury. If you prefer not to stop to stretch after warming up, be sure to stretch when you're finished exercising, while your body is still warm and flexible. See sample stretches in Chapter 6.

If you are going to run or jog, you might try warming up by walking briskly and gradually work into a run. If you're going to lift weights, do a low-level aerobic warm-up first. Then, lift weights that are light enough for you to perform numerous repetitions before moving on to heavier weights. If you're going swimming, begin with an easy slow pace at first. Then do some poolside stretches when you're finished with the aerobic portion of your workout.

When you stretch, be careful not to bounce or jerk. Bouncing might cause you to stretch beyond your limits and injure yourself. If you feel any pain, you are stretching too far. Stretching should be a pleasant sensation.

Cooling down is just as important as warming up. You need to cool down to avoid blood pooling in the legs, which could make you dizzy or cause you to faint. A cool-down time of 5 to 10 minutes should be enough.

One of the best ways to cool down is to lower the intensity of your workout during the last three to five minutes. If you've been jogging, go from a jog to a walk. Walking is a great way to cool down. After you've cooled down some but before you're ready to shower is the best time to stretch. When muscles contract during exercise, they shorten. Stretching brings the muscles back to the length they were at rest and decreases the risk of injury. Because muscles stretch a little further when they are warm, stretching during your cool down leads to improved flexibility.

DRINK PLENTY OF FLUIDS

One of the basics of safe exercise is to drink plenty of fluids, before, during, and after exercising. When you exert yourself, you will sweat. Sweating is the body's natural way of cooling itself down and getting rid of the extra heat that is generated from exercise. Even on a day you don't work out, your body loses about a liter of water cooling itself.

By sweating, you may lose up to two liters of fluid

(the amount in a large-size soft drink bottle) each hour that you exercise, depending on the temperature and humidity, the type of exercise you choose, and how hard you exercise. If you sweat off too much fluid without replacing it, you could dehydrate or suffer from over-heating (hyperthermia).

Obviously, you're in greater danger of losing too much fluid during hot months. You can avoid problems by not exercising during the hottest times of the day (even if you see others doing it). Instead, exercise early or late in the day when temperatures are more comfortable, or exercise in an air-conditioned building. By the way, it won't help you, nor is it healthy, to wear heavy clothing during warm weather to increase the amount you sweat. Sweating more won't help you lose fat weight, just water weight. You'll lose more fluid and also increase your risk of overheating.

By the time you feel thirsty, you are already becoming dehydrated. It's better to drink before you feel thirsty. Carry a water bottle with you or plan a walking route that has water fountains. You should continue to drink plenty of water throughout the day after you exercise.

Is water the best fluid replacer? In most cases, yes. If you exercise at a moderate intensity for an hour or less at moderate temperatures, drinking as much cool water as you like is the best way to keep hydrated. However, if the risk of dehydration is increased, such as in very warm weather, at high altitudes, if you're traveling a lot, or if you are active for several hours, a sports drink has some advantages.

Sports drinks provide both water and carbohydrate. The carbohydrate can be your fuel source during long workouts for which you would normally eat a snack. However, if the sports drink contains more than 10% car-

bohydrate, the water in the drink takes longer to to reach your thirsty cells. For this reason, you should choose a drink that contains 5% to 10% carbohydrate, which moves about as fast as water into the cells. Drinks with more than 10% carbohydrate, such as some sports drinks, fruit juice, and regular sodas, should be mixed half and half with water before drinking. Despite the hype, you don't usually need to worry about finding a drink that contains sodium, potassium, chloride, and magnesium (unless you're an endurance sports athlete or exercise in hot weather). A healthy diet provides enough of these minerals to replace the amount lost through sweat.

If you have a heart problem or are on a fluid-restricted diet, talk with your doctor about what to do to keep a balanced fluid level during exercise.

KEEPING ONE FOOT AHEAD OF PROBLEMS

Now let's talk about your feet. People with diabetes are at risk of having poor circulation in their feet. (However, regular exercise helps improve foot circulation.) And they are at risk for neuropathy (nerve damage). Poor circulation prevents foot tissues from fighting infections. Neuropathy often prevents a person from feeling injuries to the feet. Before you start an exercise program, have your ability to feel sensation in your feet tested.

It is important to check your feet daily and before and after you exercise. Blisters on your feet mean you overdid it. You're looking for any redness, swelling, or warm skin temperature that indicate inflammation. Opened blisters, cuts, or scratches on your feet could lead to an infection. Where your feet are concerned, things can go from bad to worse very quickly. Ask your health-care team ahead of time how you should treat blisters or other foot wounds.

For blisters, cuts, athlete's foot, and calluses, follow the treatment instructions of your health-care team. Because you have diabetes, these conditions need special attention. Ignoring them is a big mistake. Most podiatrists will tell you that you can make problems even worse by trying "home surgery." Don't break any blisters that develop. If you see redness indicating inflammation, talk to your doctor or podiatrist. Persistent redness or swelling, with or without pain, needs immediate professional attention. Don't try to treat these problems without the advice of your health-care team.

To avoid these nasty irritations,

- choose well-fitting shoes
- choose shoes that are designed for the exercise you're planning (in other words, don't jog in shoes that are designed for tennis)
- always start your exercise in clean, smooth-fitting socks.

When choosing shoes, take the time to get a perfect fit. This may mean getting help from a shoe-fitting professional. More than 80 percent of all the shoes sold in the United States are imported, which means that a size you've chosen for one shoe might not be the right size in every shoe. So try different sizes in different styles.

If you have trouble finding shoes that fit your feet, you will benefit from professional advice. This is critical if you've lost sensation in your feet, because you can't trust the way a shoe feels, and you will need professional help to determine proper fit. Podiatrists are trained in footwear design and modification, but most shoe salespeople are not. Stores that specialize in prescription footwear will probably have on staff a pedorthist, a specialist trained in fitting shoes for people with painful or disabling foot conditions.

You can choose which shoes to try on by first looking at the shape of your foot and selecting a style that most closely matches your foot shape. For example, if your foot is broad at the toes, a shoe tapered at the toe won't be a good choice. If your foot is straight with a flattened arch, you won't want a shoe that curves in at the instep toward the middle of the shoe. A shoe should not put any pressure on your toes from the top or sides. Some people think they can get more room for their toes by choosing a wider sized shoe. But a wider shoe won't do the trick: it will just be too loose. Feel around inside the shoes with your hand for any rough spots or overlapping seams that may cause blisters or cuts. Make sure your new shoes won't injure your feet by wearing them several times before using them as your full-time exercise shoes.

For the best fit, you should measure both feet. Most people have one foot longer than the other. When trying on shoes, wear the socks you intend to use for exercise. Lace them up and evaluate the fit while standing. A shoe should be 1/2 to 5/8 inch (about a finger's width) longer than the longest toe. Fit the shoes to the longest foot.

A shoe that is too loose will rub on your foot as you walk and cause blisters. Some people put insoles in their shoes to improve the cushion or to keep the shoe from slipping. Be careful not to choose too thick of an insole, because it can make the shoe too tight. Many people get benefits from shoe inserts designed specifically for their feet, called orthotics. Orthotic inserts are shaped to help favorably distribute your body weight across the bottom of the foot. These should be prescribed. If needed, your podiatrist will determine the beneficial design and have them made. They can be expensive; however, they may make the difference in your ability to stay active.

The final test is to move around in the shoes in much the same way that you would for the exercise you're going to be doing. Walk or jog in them. Move from side to side.

- Do the shoes feel comfortable?
- Do your feet feel supported but not squeezed?
- Do you feel cushioning in the heel and forefoot?
- Can you feel anything rubbing your foot or causing pressure on any part of your foot?
- Does your heel stay put and not slip when you walk or jog? If the heel is too big or too tight, you could be surprised with some painful blisters after you exercise.
- Check your toes. Do they push against the front end of the shoe? If so, you need a larger size.

Choose a good pair of socks, too. Exercise in socks that are made all or mostly of absorbent natural fibers, such as wool or cotton. Make sure they fit well and don't have creases, wrinkles, or holes that could irritate your foot as you exercise. And always start your exercise in a clean pair of socks. Dirty socks are an invitation for foot infection.

After hunting for the right pair of shoes, remember that shoes wear out. Worn out shoes stop giving you all the advantages that were advertised when you bought them. They also increase your chances of an exercise injury. How fast your shoes wear out depends on how much you use them. One guideline is to replace your shoes every six months, or about every 400 miles.

DRESS FOR THE WEATHER

The clothes you wear are important, too. They should fit the weather. If the temperature is cold, dress in layers of loose-fitting clothes. As you get hot, you can take off a layer and tie it around your waist; it will be convenient to put back on while you cool down.

For cold weather layering, it's best to choose something made of polypropylene, silk, or thin, fine wool for the first layer. These materials help lift perspiration from your body to be evaporated. For the middle layer, choose something made of knitted wool or synthetic pile. On the outside, wear a windbreaker made of material that will breathe and allow perspiration to escape. During the day, choose dark clothing that will absorb the heat from the sun. Wear gloves and a hat or hood to protect you from the cold. If the weather is too severe (a windchill of 15° fahrenheit or lower) stay inside.

If you're exercising outside at night, choose something brightly colored and reflective.

If it's hot outside, you'll want to wear as little as you can. The best clothing for hot weather is made of a fabric, such as cotton, that is light, will breathe, and allows perspiration to evaporate. Stay clear of clothing made of rubber or plastic because they trap heat and moisture and prevent your body from cooling down.

Consider exercise clothes made of a cotton/spandex or lycra mixture, which will gently support your body, much like "support" hose. Because they hug your body, there are no loose clothing folds to chafe your skin. Moving in them feels a little easier. ❧

CHAPTER 6

Exercising to Increase Your *Fitness*

FITNESS HAS FOUR COMPONENTS: CARDIOVASCULAR OR AEROBIC FITNESS, MUSCLE STRENGTH AND ENDURANCE, BODY FLEXIBILITY, AND BODY COMPOSITION. An exercise program that increases your healthfulness in all these areas will give you the best results.

GETTING AEROBICALLY FIT

Aerobic activities increase fitness by building the ability of the heart, lungs, and circulatory system to supply oxygen and nutrients effectively to working muscles. As you become aerobically fit, your body will work more efficiently, you'll have more energy, you should lose weight, and you'll be able to perform your exercises and other activities without running out of breath as easily.

With regular workouts, your body adapts to the demands of aerobic exercise. Your heart will get stronger as you get more fit. During exercise, your heart needs to pump more blood with each beat. Your arteries become dilated so that more blood can be carried to your muscles. The expanded volume of blood going through the heart supplies the muscles with blood, and the muscles become more efficient at absorbing oxygen from the blood and in converting stored fats and carbohydrates into energy. Over time, aerobic exercise will lead to an improvement in your VO_2 max (see Chapter 4).

One improvement you won't need exercise testing to measure will be in your resting heart rate. You can determine it by just comparing your resting heart rate (your heart rate when you are not exercising) with that of what it was several months before you began exercising. (Don't be tempted to compare heart rates with someone else—heart rate range is largely determined genetically; another person's heart rate may be a lot slower or faster than yours without corrresponding to fitness.) A lower resting heart rate will indicate that your heart is processing the same amount of blood with less effort than it did when you were less fit. To measure your heart rate, count your wrist or neck pulse for a full minute while you are sitting down.

If you want to get fit aerobically, you should participate in exercises that are aerobic. Aerobic by definition means that you need to exercise at least three times a week, and each of those exercise sessions need to be at least 20 minutes of sustained exercise. Stop and go activities such as baseball and golfing with a cart don't cut it. Some sports, such as tennis or basketball can be aerobic, depending on how actively you play them (but typically there is too much stopping in these sports to be aerobic). Even lifting weights can be aerobic, for instance, with circuit weight training (performing exercises that work large muscle groups and moving quickly from one exercise to another with short rest periods).

Walking.

If you're just beginning an aerobic exercise program, there couldn't be a better exercise. In fact, walking is gaining popularity among even the hardiest exercisers. One of the attractions to walking is that the risk of injury is extremely low—you don't get the orthopedic (skeletal) impact in each step that you do with running. You don't have to learn any new skills—you know how to walk. The trick, however, is to get your heart rate up. If you're in good shape, a leisurely stroll won't give you much of an aerobic workout. But if you've been sedentary, this may be a good workout for you. The point is that you need to walk at a pace that will give you a workout but won't be too hard for you. A good rule of thumb is to walk at a pace that is quick but at which you can carry on a conversation.

How long should you walk? If you're just starting out, you might only be able to walk for a few minutes without getting fatigued. You should gradually work up to walking for 45 minutes, three to five days a week. Build up your time by adding three to five minutes each week over many weeks. By adding duration (the length of time you walk) to your walks instead of intensity (how fast you walk), you can safely progress in your workouts.

When you begin, try walking at a pace that is comfortable but in which you do get up to your target heart rate (for more on heart rates, see Chapter 4). As you get in shape and you're able to walk for the full amount of time, you may have trouble reaching your target heart rate. You may want to try increasing the length of your stride and the number of steps you take a minute. As you get in even better shape, it might get harder to quicken your steps. To improve your workout, choose a route that has more hills. But don't take that route too soon.

Equipment needed: Comfortable clothes (extra fabric between your legs could lead to chafing—choose close-fitting shorts or pants to protect your skin, which can be worn alone or under baggy pants) and a good pair of walking shoes fitted while wearing exercise socks (see Chapter 5).

Running/jogging.

These are both good forms of aerobic exercise, but they put you at risk for injury. When you run, your feet hit the ground some 800 to 2,000 times a mile. Each time they hit the ground, your feet and legs get a jolt of about three to five times your body weight. No wonder that running injuries do happen. Most of these injuries happen to the joints, ligaments, and muscles of the lower body. Guidelines for avoiding injury are to rest your body between runs (by running every other day)

and to stick to a routine of warming up and gentle stretching before you run and cooling down and gentle stretching afterward.

If you feel pain while running, slow down to a walk until the pain goes away. If you feel it again as you begin to run, stop again and give your feet and legs a rest for a few days. If the pain persists, see your doctor. Preventing some injuries might be as simple as changing the length of your stride, your speed, or the way your foot strikes the ground. An exercise physiologist can help you find the best stride for you. You can lessen the risk by running on softer surfaces, such as a wood-chip or dirt trail. Concrete (typical sidewalks) is the worst surface to run on. You should also choose a good pair of running shoes that have plenty of cushion to ease the blow each time your feet hit the ground.

If you've never run before or haven't run for a long time, you should first be able to walk two miles within 30 minutes without breathing hard. If you can do this, try alternating running with walking every five minutes. Do this for the first three to four weeks of your program and gradually increase the time that you run. Don't be tempted to run too far too quickly. Stay within your target heart rate. If you can carry on a conversation while you run, you're doing fine. Run for time, not mileage. Sticking to your goal to run for 20 to 45 minutes instead of running a long distance will keep you from the temptation of overdoing it.

Equipment needed: Comfortable, nonchafing clothing, a supportive bra or athletic supporter, and well-cushioned running shoes.

Swimming.

One real benefit of swimming is that the risk for

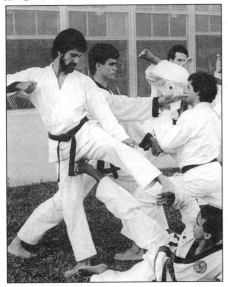

"IT WAS SCARY BEING DIAGNOSED WITH DIABETES."

For some, exercise is inextricably woven into the fabric of daily life. Rick Cabrera, an exercise physiologist from Coral Gables, Florida, has practiced Tae Kwon Do since he was 12. A Korean martial art, Tae Kwon Do literally translates as "the art of hands and feet." Now 33, Rick says Tae Kwon Do enhances his life mentally, spiritually, and physically. "I've been doing it for so long, I don't look at it as a sport. If I really wanted to play a game for pure entertainment, I would go out for a pick-up game of basketball or hit the gym. The martial arts go beyond that. Even though you practice Tae Kwon Do in a physical sense, every physical move has to do with the spirit and the mind. A lot of what you do in practice sessions, you use in your daily life."

Just how does Tae Kwon Do help with the stresses and strains of everyday life? Rick says recalling his state of mind during practice sessions helps him cope. He also says his martial arts practice helps his diabetes control. When an occasional high blood glucose reading crops up, instead of focusing on negative thoughts, Rick tries to recapture his state of mind during practice. For him, it's a calming influence.

Rick was diagnosed with type I diabetes 12 years ago, during his last semester of college. Not only was the diagnosis a shock—there was no family history of the disease—but controlling his blood glucose levels was a problem. "I had to drop out that last semester to try to get everything under control," Rick recalls. At first, he relied on the college health service for treatment, but not getting the level of care he needed, he went home. There an endocrinologist helped get him on the right track. That summer, he returned to the University of Florida and finished up his degree in exercise physiology.

Rick had played basketball since high school, and his first jobs out of college were coaching high school teams. His love of Tae Kwon Do continued, but it seemed as though diabetes would put a stop to competing. "My biggest downfall was when I traveled to areas where they held the competitions. They never went on schedule, and I never knew exactly when I'd be competing. We were there from nine in the morning." Rick remembers the frustration of trying to regulate his food intake for the day and adjust his insulin under such uncertain conditions. "I remember experiencing some pretty bad reactions and some pretty high readings," he says.

Another worry: Tae Kwon Do, a very traditional sport, is practiced barefooted. In fact, foot injury is a serious concern for Rick. "Sometimes I go on some pretty rough floors. I can get blisters, and the impact on my feet when practicing is tough. That's always been a big concern for me. It was a scary thing being diagnosed with diabetes. The first thing that ran through my mind was, 'There it is. I can't do this any more.' I knew that people with diabetes can develop foot problems, and there was a chance of amputation."

Accepting the risks, Rick continues to practice Tae Kwon Do barefooted. As a safety precaution, he uses a spray called Second Skin on his feet for a slight bit of protection and wears foam shinguards that cover his shin and instep. "If there should be some injury, I tend to it as quickly as I can and lay off training until it heals." Rick also checks with his physician immediately if an injury occurs.

Today, Rick works as an exercise physiologist with the Diabetes Fitness Program of the Health and Fitness Institute at Doctors Hospital in Coral Gables, Florida. Rick develops exercise programs for people with diabetes and helps monitor their progress as they move into fitness. Putting his muscle where his mouth is, Rick's typical exercise routine consists of weight training on Monday, Wednesday, and Friday, with a Tae Kwon Do practice in the evenings. On Tuesday and Thursday, he concentrates on aerobic conditioning, running or doing some other form of aerobic exercise, with a second evening workout. Saturday morning is devoted to a two-hour plus Tae Kwon Do practice, and Sunday he takes a day off.

Even though exercise is an integral part of Rick's life, he hasn't lost the ability to relate to those for whom exercise is a dirty word. When he works with patients, he tries to encourage them to gently incorporate more activity into their own lives. "When you increase your activity level, you're basically exercising," he says.

After briefing a patient on the scientific and medical reasons why exercise is good medicine, he advises, "Let's try to find something that's enjoyable to you. Something that you've been doing your whole life that you already enjoy, such as going to the mall. You enjoy going to the mall; you're

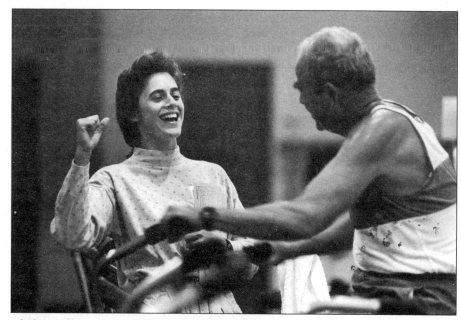

It helps to have support from those around you.
Photograph by Les Todd, courtesy of Duke University Photo Department.

walking. Let's just add to this. You'll walk in the mall three times a week and monitor your pulse rate." Rick says, "People newly diagnosed with diabetes already have a lot of lifestyle changes that they're having to make. I think about how I can make that a little easier and help them realize that exercise can be a part of their lives." ■

injury is extremely low. One of the main drawbacks of swimming is that you need a pool (or lake or ocean) to do it—so there could be some expense involved. Swimming is a great way to get aerobically fit. If you're a swimming novice, it will take some time getting coordinated enough with your swimming technique to get a good workout. Swimming with a kick board is an easy way to start a swimming program.

At first, begin by swimming two or four laps and rest between each set of laps. Then swim more laps and rest again. As you get in shape, increase the number of laps you swim and shorten the rest period. A technique that many swimmers use is called a pyramid. They begin by swimming one lap, rest, swim two laps, rest, swim three laps, rest and so on until they get to eight laps. Then they reverse the order by swimming eight laps and resting, swimming seven laps and resting, and so on until they get to the last lap. This will give you a good workout, but you should only try it once you get in better shape.

Don't think a pool workout only means swimming laps! There are lots of ways to exercise in water. For instance, you can join an aqua aerobics class. This is for you if you're not a "swimmer." You don't even need to know how to swim to participate in most classes—but you do need to feel comfortable in water. In one type of workout, you wear a flotation belt and never touch the bottom of the pool. Some classes include stretching and toning, using the water as resistance.

Another activity that uses the water's resistance for a good aerobic workout is water walking. The water height should be between your waist and underarms. If the pool water level allows it, walk the pool end-to-end or in a serpentine pattern, or walk from side to side—

forward, backward, or sideways. For every lap you walk forward, walk another one backward. Don't forget to use your arms: you can do a traditional swimming stroke motion such as breast stroke or other movements such as alternating biceps curls.

Equipment needed: A swimsuit and foot guards (like Aquasocks) to protect your feet from injury on the sides or bottom of the pool, lake, or ocean. You may also want swimming goggles to protect your eyes from the pool's chlorine.

Aerobic dance.

Aerobic dance combines choreographed exercise with music. A lot of people (it's not just for women) like aerobic dance because it is less boring than other exercises. You get to meet other people, and there are numerous routines and invigorating music to keep it interesting. The fact that you're using both your arms and your legs to exercise makes aerobic dance equal to running in terms of burning calories and getting aerobically fit.

The risk for injury depends on your level of fitness, the expertise of the instructor, and the quality of the floor and your shoes. High-impact aerobics involves some jumping up and down movements (like jumping jacks) and adding some bounce to your routines. Low-impact aerobics relies more on upper body movements and moving from foot to foot without giving an extra bounce.

Step or bench aerobics involves stepping gently up onto and off of a bench. Benches have adjustable heights. Starting out, you'll want to try the lowest height until you have confidence in where you are placing your feet. Feet should step entirely onto the bench, with no part of the foot hanging off the edge. Most benches start at about 4 inches in height and can be adjusted in 2- to 3 inch increments. As you become aerobically fit, you can add more risers to increase bench height.

You'll need a good pair of aerobic shoes. They are designed for the side-to-side movement and have cushioning in parts of the shoe that take the most shock. Don't try to do these exercises in running shoes. Running shoes are designed only for forward movement. Look for socks that have extra padding along the bottoms, especially on the ball and heel areas, for added comfort.

Make sure that the floor you're exercising on has some cushion to it. Most aerobics studios have wooden floors or floors constructed especially for aerobics that give when body weight comes down with some force. The floor surface should not be slippery. A concrete floor will be hard on your ankles and knees, so choose carefully where you set up your VCR if you're working out at home.

When starting out, ease into the routine. You don't have to work out at the same level of those in the class—which you might be tempted to do. A good aerobics instructor will remind you to work at your own pace. Lift your legs or arms only half as high as the instructor does. Don't try to keep the same pace as others, and rest by walking or marching in place if your heart rate is going too high. Join in again when you're ready, and don't forget to stop for water whenever you need it. As you build up endurance, increase the time you spend doing the routines.

Equipment needed: Comfortable clothes that allow free arm and leg movements and well-cushioned aerobic shoes.

Bicycling.

Even people who think exercise is pure drudgery discover that they love to ride a bike for fitness. The risk for injury from the exercise itself is low because your weight is carried by the bicycle and is not placed on your body.

Bicycling has its drawbacks. Bikes can be expensive. And finding a trail on which you can ride without being interrupted by frequent traffic lights can be difficult. But overall, bicycling is a great workout.

To begin, choose a route that is fairly level with few hills and pedal in the low (lowest resistance, easiest to pedal) to moderate gears of your bike. As you get in shape, increase your pedaling speed and choose more challenging routes. You can also increase the resistance against which you pedal, but add resistance cautiously. Because this makes it harder to pedal, it puts added strain on your muscles and tendons. Always check your target heart rate to be sure you're not pedalling too hard.

When buying a bike, take the time to get a correct fit. When the ball of your foot is on the pedal, your leg should be only slightly flexed. But you should not have to wobble from side to side as you reach down to pedal. Choosing a bike that makes you lean slightly forward as you pedal will mean you'll have the opportunity to really shape up your gluteal (buttock) muscles, and your arms will also have to work to support some of your weight as you lean on them. Shop around and talk to many bike shop employees about what might be right for you. Look into buying an ultracomfortable gel bike seat, so you'll look forward to your rides.

Equipment needed: A bicycle and a helmet.

Cross-country skiing.

Spending a winter day outside is a delightful experience. Cross-country skiing involves gliding instead of bouncing, so the risk for impact injury is low. And it works both the upper and lower body. The one drawback is that you need snow (unless you do it inside on a machine, of course). This exercise requires skill, balance, and good arm and leg coordination. Even if you're in good shape, it will take practice to perform this exercise properly. This full-body exercise can be wonderfully exhausting.

If you're a beginner, start by exercising in just the skis without the poles on flat, level ground. Take short steps and then glide. Once you get good at a skiing stride, add the poles so that both your arms and legs are working to move you along. Gradually speed up your movement and work on technique. Also, begin to tackle uphill grades. Because technique is difficult to grasp at first, you'd benefit by taking a few lessons.

Equipment needed: Skis, poles, boots, and layers of warm clothing or a cross-country skiing machine. If you're going outside, carry a fanny pack with snacks and blood-testing supplies.

STRENGTH TRAINING

Aerobic exercise is great for building up the heart and lungs. But it is limited in building your muscles—especially if you focus on just one exercise. For example, if all you do is run, your legs will get toned and strengthened, but your upper body will be missing out.

The sad fact about getting older is that our bodies naturally lose muscle mass—especially if we don't use them. The only way to preserve and to build muscle mass and strength is to work your muscles against some kind of resistance. The best way to develop muscle strength and increase endurance is through resistance or weight training. This involves lifting, pushing, or pulling weights.

There are several ways to become fit with resistance training. One way is with free weights. Free weights are barbells and dumbbells. When you lift barbells or dumbbells, the weight of the bar remains the same. Another way to lift weights is by using a machine that has a weight stack attached to a cable or chain and a pulley. On some machines, the pulley or cam is off-center. On these machines, the weights get lighter or heavier depending on the position of the cam. Other forms of resistance training include working out with large elastic bands or springs and using your body as resistance with calisthenics such as sit ups, push ups, and pull ups.

See the accompanying sample exercises for strengthening important muscle groups. The handheld weights can be barbells or dumbbells or even small soup cans that you can grip comfortably.

An advantage of working out on weight machines is that you can exercise alone. For some exercises with free weights, you need someone to spot you—to be with you as you lift and help you lift the weight off your body if you are unable.

Depending on your goals, you may choose to work out with free weights or weight machines or by doing calisthenics. Some people believe that free weights are better because you have to balance the bar and therefore use more muscles to lift the bar. The truth is that whichever choice you make, you'll benefit greatly in terms of increasing strength and muscle mass.

You should work with an exercise physiologist, a

STRENGTHENING EXERCISES

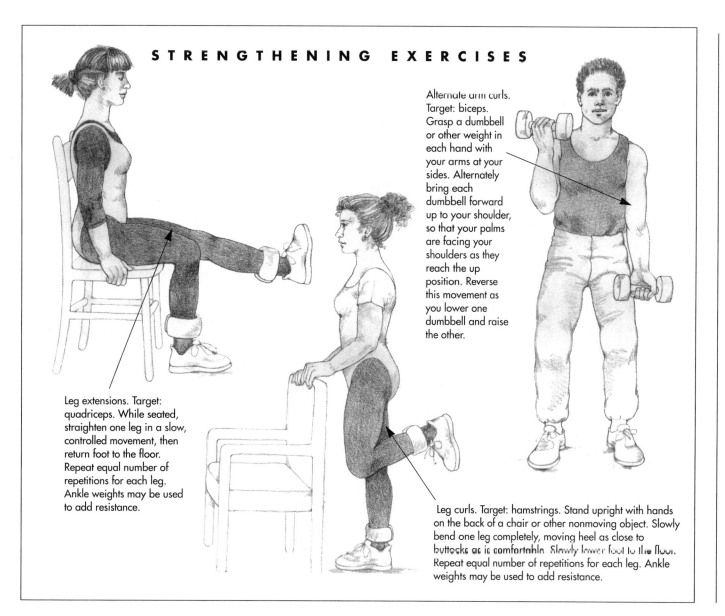

Alternate arm curls. Target: biceps. Grasp a dumbbell or other weight in each hand with your arms at your sides. Alternately bring each dumbbell forward up to your shoulder, so that your palms are facing your shoulders as they reach the up position. Reverse this movement as you lower one dumbbell and raise the other.

Leg extensions. Target: quadriceps. While seated, straighten one leg in a slow, controlled movement, then return foot to the floor. Repeat equal number of repetitions for each leg. Ankle weights may be used to add resistance.

Leg curls. Target: hamstrings. Stand upright with hands on the back of a chair or other nonmoving object. Slowly bend one leg completely, moving heel as close to buttocks as is comfortable. Slowly lower foot to the floor. Repeat equal number of repetitions for each leg. Ankle weights may be used to add resistance.

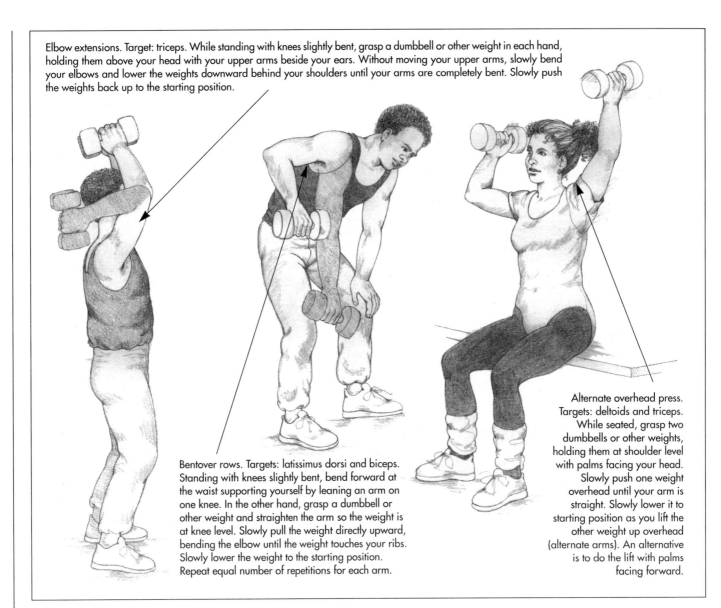

Elbow extensions. Target: triceps. While standing with knees slightly bent, grasp a dumbbell or other weight in each hand, holding them above your head with your upper arms beside your ears. Without moving your upper arms, slowly bend your elbows and lower the weights downward behind your shoulders until your arms are completely bent. Slowly push the weights back up to the starting position.

Bentover rows. Targets: latissimus dorsi and biceps. Standing with knees slightly bent, bend forward at the waist supporting yourself by leaning an arm on one knee. In the other hand, grasp a dumbbell or other weight and straighten the arm so the weight is at knee level. Slowly pull the weight directly upward, bending the elbow until the weight touches your ribs. Slowly lower the weight to the starting position. Repeat equal number of repetitions for each arm.

Alternate overhead press. Targets: deltoids and triceps. While seated, grasp two dumbbells or other weights, holding them at shoulder level with palms facing your head. Slowly push one weight overhead until your arm is straight. Slowly lower it to starting position as you lift the other weight up overhead (alternate arms). An alternative is to do the lift with palms facing forward.

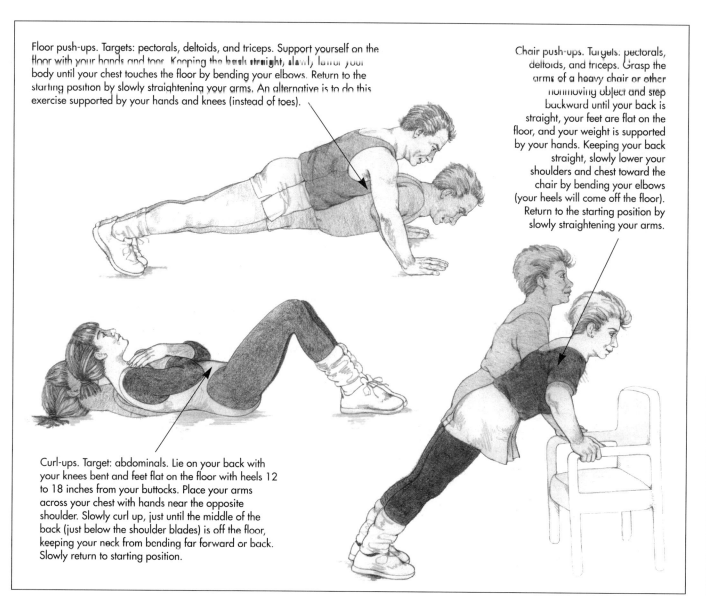

Floor push-ups. Targets: pectorals, deltoids, and triceps. Support yourself on the floor with your hands and toes. Keeping the back straight, slowly lower your body until your chest touches the floor by bending your elbows. Return to the starting position by slowly straightening your arms. An alternative is to do this exercise supported by your hands and knees (instead of toes).

Chair push-ups. Targets: pectorals, deltoids, and triceps. Grasp the arms of a heavy chair or other nonmoving object and step backward until your back is straight, your feet are flat on the floor, and your weight is supported by your hands. Keeping your back straight, slowly lower your shoulders and chest toward the chair by bending your elbows (your heels will come off the floor). Return to the starting position by slowly straightening your arms.

Curl-ups. Target: abdominals. Lie on your back with your knees bent and feet flat on the floor with heels 12 to 18 inches from your buttocks. Place your arms across your chest with hands near the opposite shoulder. Slowly curl up, just until the middle of the back (just below the shoulder blades) is off the floor, keeping your neck from bending far forward or back. Slowly return to starting position.

certified strength and conditioning specialist (trained and certified by the National Strength and Conditioning Association; see Resources), or some other exercise specialist to show you the correct and safe way to lift weights. Learning and using the correct form is important for you to gain the full benefit of each lift and to prevent injury. To help, here are a few tips when lifting weights.

- Warm up before you lift to increase body temperature and blood flow. You can begin by doing some light calisthenics or 5 to 10 minutes of aerobic exercise such as riding an exercise bicycle or walking. After you are warmed up, do some stretching exercises. Also, start by lifting some light weights before going on to conquer heavier weights.
- Breathe properly during each lift. Don't hold your breath when you lift a weight. Doing so can cause your blood pressure to go too high and make you dizzy or faint. Breathe in as you lower the weight and breathe out as you lift.
- Learn how to use the equipment and how to lift properly before you start to work out.
- Don't expect fast results. It takes time before you see real results in the mirror. This is especially true if you have a lot of body fat. The fat will hide the muscles you're working so hard to build. Although you might not see great results at first, you will feel them in terms of better endurance, greater energy to do ordinary things such as household chores, and to lift even heavier weights.
- Take a day off between workouts. Your muscles need adequate rest to get stronger. It usually takes about 48 hours for your muscles to recover from strenuous exercise. So, you should not lift more often than every other day. Some weight lifters work on the upper body one day and the lower body the next, resting them on alternate days.

ACTIVITIES TO IMPROVE FLEXIBILITY

What is flexibility? Basically it means how far you can stretch your muscles around their joints comfortably. Flexibility is often measured as a range of motion that you are able to perform. The more flexible you are, the more you can stretch your muscles. Flexibility helps to decrease the tension on your muscles. This helps you prevent injuries not only while exercising but also in daily life. Flexible people move comfortably in all situations.

The best way to gain flexibility is to do stretching exercises daily. If you haven't stretched for some time, don't expect rapid results. For instance, it may take months before you are able to touch your toes. In fact, you may never be able to bend over and touch your toes. But you can get a lot closer!

Whenever you stretch, go slowly, breathe evenly, and do not bounce. Make each stretch a smooth, careful movement. Only stretch so far that you don't feel pain. If you feel pain, you are stretching too far. Let your body tell you how far you should stretch. (Note that if you have peripheral neuropathy, you may not be able to feel yourself overstretching.) Each of us has different limits. If you stretch too far, you can injure yourself.

Stretch to a comfortable point, hold for at least 8 to 10 seconds (you may work up to 30 seconds or more) while continuing to breathe, and release. Don't strain!

STRETCHING EXERCISES

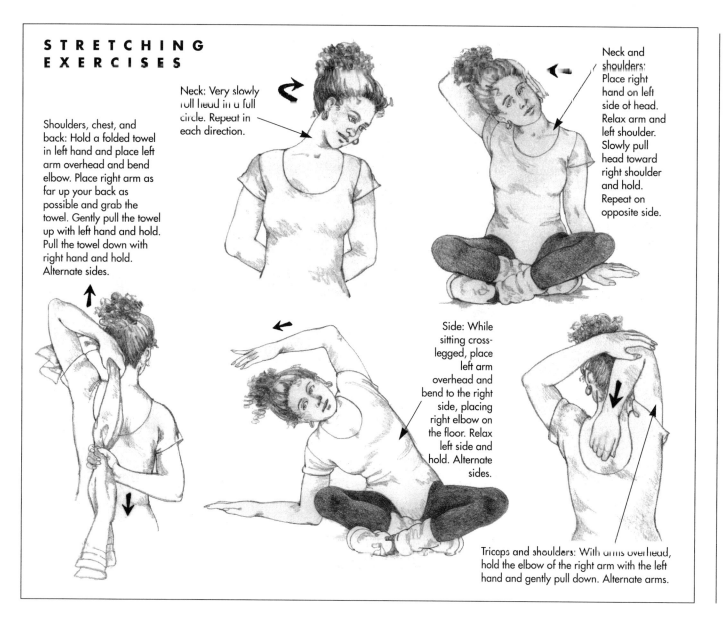

Shoulders, chest, and back: Hold a folded towel in left hand and place left arm overhead and bend elbow. Place right arm as far up your back as possible and grab the towel. Gently pull the towel up with left hand and hold. Pull the towel down with right hand and hold. Alternate sides.

Neck: Very slowly roll head in a full circle. Repeat in each direction.

Neck and shoulders: Place right hand on left side of head. Relax arm and left shoulder. Slowly pull head toward right shoulder and hold. Repeat on opposite side.

Side: While sitting cross-legged, place left arm overhead and bend to the right side, placing right elbow on the floor. Relax left side and hold. Alternate sides.

Triceps and shoulders: With arms overhead, hold the elbow of the right arm with the left hand and gently pull down. Alternate arms.

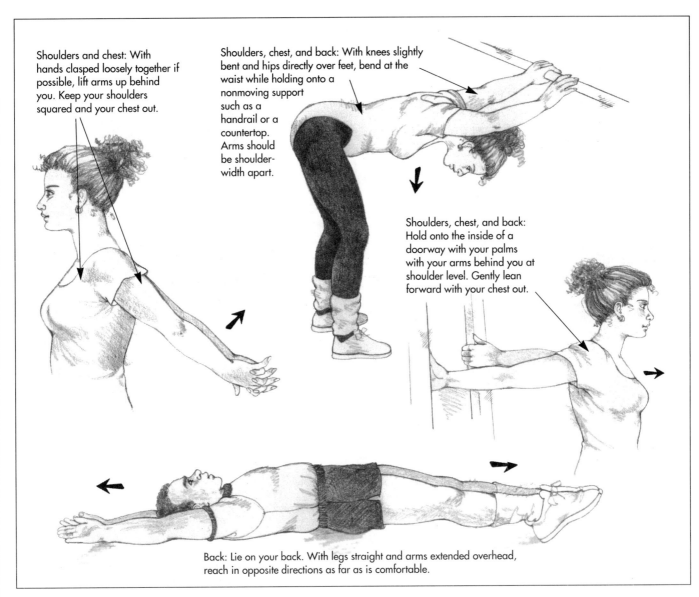

Shoulders and chest: With hands clasped loosely together if possible, lift arms up behind you. Keep your shoulders squared and your chest out.

Shoulders, chest, and back: With knees slightly bent and hips directly over feet, bend at the waist while holding onto a nonmoving support such as a handrail or a countertop. Arms should be shoulder-width apart.

Shoulders, chest, and back: Hold onto the inside of a doorway with your palms with your arms behind you at shoulder level. Gently lean forward with your chest out.

Back: Lie on your back. With legs straight and arms extended overhead, reach in opposite directions as far as is comfortable.

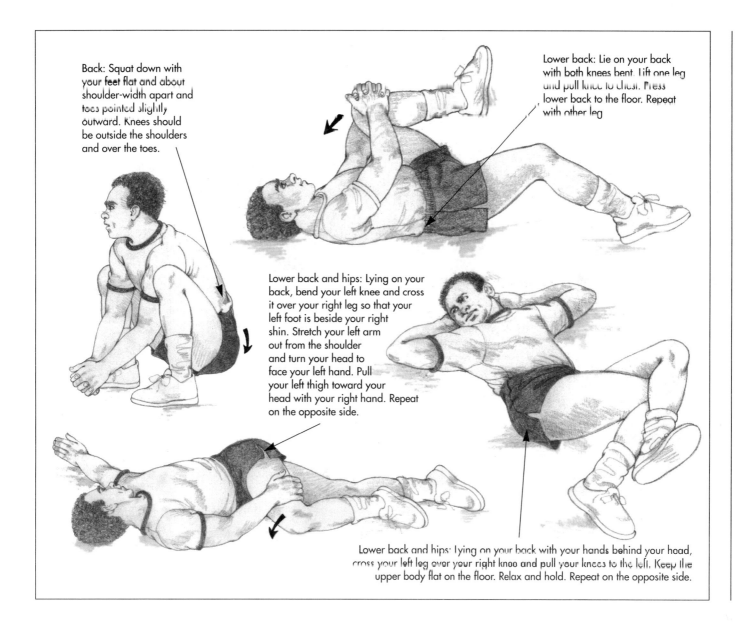

Back: Squat down with your feet flat and about shoulder-width apart and toes pointed slightly outward. Knees should be outside the shoulders and over the toes.

Lower back: Lie on your back with both knees bent. Lift one leg and pull knee to chest. Press lower back to the floor. Repeat with other leg

Lower back and hips: Lying on your back, bend your left knee and cross it over your right leg so that your left foot is beside your right shin. Stretch your left arm out from the shoulder and turn your head to face your left hand. Pull your left thigh toward your head with your right hand. Repeat on the opposite side.

Lower back and hips: Lying on your back with your hands behind your head, cross your left leg over your right knee and pull your knees to the left. Keep the upper body flat on the floor. Relax and hold. Repeat on the opposite side.

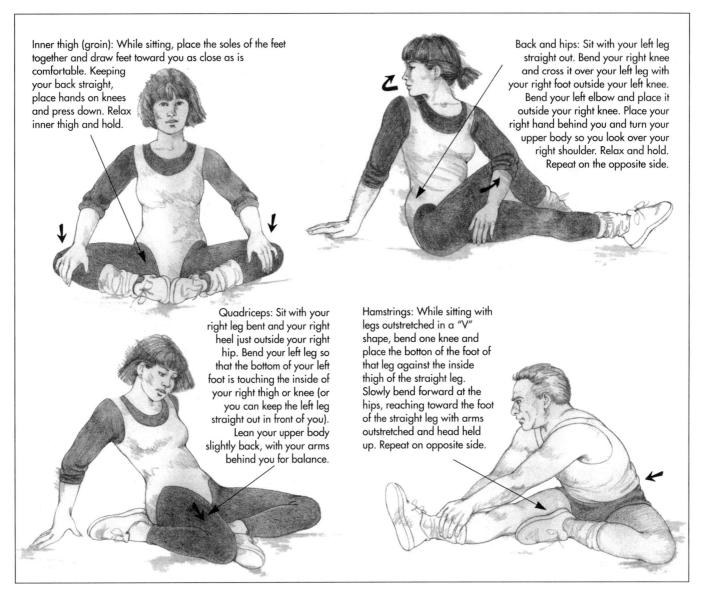

Inner thigh (groin): While sitting, place the soles of the feet together and draw feet toward you as close as is comfortable. Keeping your back straight, place hands on knees and press down. Relax inner thigh and hold.

Back and hips: Sit with your left leg straight out. Bend your right knee and cross it over your left leg with your right foot outside your left knee. Bend your left elbow and place it outside your right knee. Place your right hand behind you and turn your upper body so you look over your right shoulder. Relax and hold. Repeat on the opposite side.

Quadriceps: Sit with your right leg bent and your right heel just outside your right hip. Bend your left leg so that the bottom of your left foot is touching the inside of your right thigh or knee (or you can keep the left leg straight out in front of you). Lean your upper body slightly back, with your arms behind you for balance.

Hamstrings: While sitting with legs outstretched in a "V" shape, bend one knee and place the bottom of the foot of that leg against the inside thigh of the straight leg. Slowly bend forward at the hips, reaching toward the foot of the straight leg with arms outstretched and head held up. Repeat on opposite side.

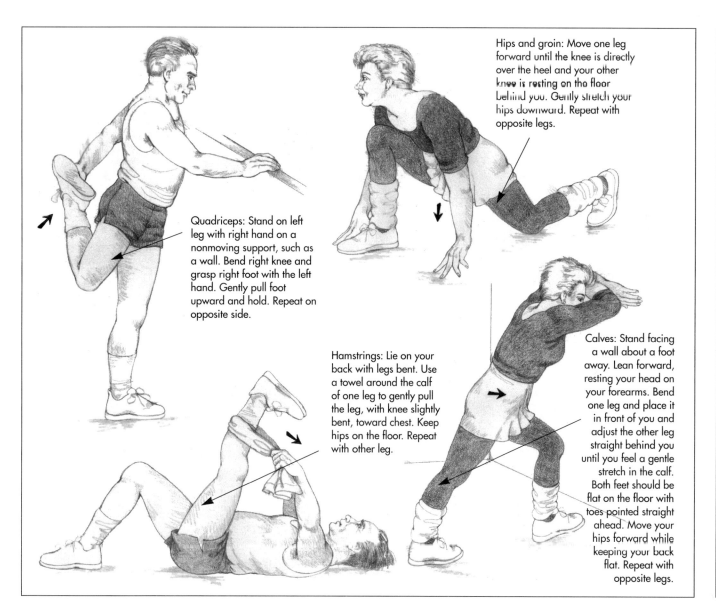

Quadriceps: Stand on left leg with right hand on a nonmoving support, such as a wall. Bend right knee and grasp right foot with the left hand. Gently pull foot upward and hold. Repeat on opposite side.

Hips and groin: Move one leg forward until the knee is directly over the heel and your other knee is resting on the floor behind you. Gently stretch your hips downward. Repeat with opposite legs.

Hamstrings: Lie on your back with legs bent. Use a towel around the calf of one leg to gently pull the leg, with knee slightly bent, toward chest. Keep hips on the floor. Repeat with other leg.

Calves: Stand facing a wall about a foot away. Lean forward, resting your head on your forearms. Bend one leg and place it in front of you and adjust the other leg straight behind you until you feel a gentle stretch in the calf. Both feet should be flat on the floor with toes pointed straight ahead. Move your hips forward while keeping your back flat. Repeat with opposite legs.

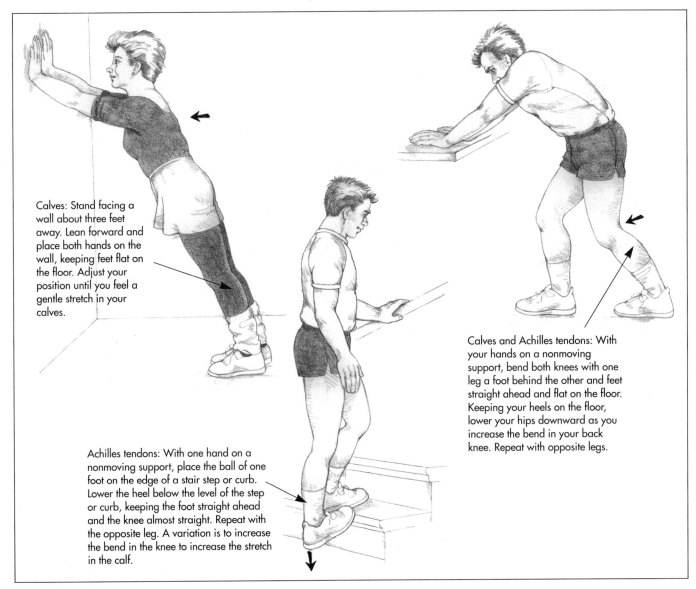

Calves: Stand facing a wall about three feet away. Lean forward and place both hands on the wall, keeping feet flat on the floor. Adjust your position until you feel a gentle stretch in your calves.

Achilles tendons: With one hand on a nonmoving support, place the ball of one foot on the edge of a stair step or curb. Lower the heel below the level of the step or curb, keeping the foot straight ahead and the knee almost straight. Repeat with the opposite leg. A variation is to increase the bend in the knee to increase the stretch in the calf.

Calves and Achilles tendons: With your hands on a nonmoving support, bend both knees with one leg a foot behind the other and feet straight ahead and flat on the floor. Keeping your heels on the floor, lower your hips downward as you increase the bend in your back knee. Repeat with opposite legs.

Think about relaxing each of the muscles as you stretch them. Try to perform each stretch several times slowly. Do stretches that focus on all the major muscle groups These groups include your neck, shoulders, chest, lower back, hips, inner thigh (groin), hamstrings, and calves. See the accompanying sample stretches for various parts of your body. Before or after each workout, be sure to stretch those muscles that you will use or did use in your regular exercise routine.

A yoga class or VCR tape can help you take stretching to new heights of enjoyment. Yoga involves holding your body in various positions or during a series of slow movements while you concentrate on your breathing patterns. Yoga improves your flexibility and increases your strength and energy, and you may even find relief from both physical and mental stress. There are different kinds of yoga (some more active or meditative than others), so ask a lot of questions while you figure out which type will suit you.

The advantage of attending a class rather than using a tape is that the teacher will correct your body positions so you get the best results. Yoga is an excellent way to exercise if you haven't been active for a while, if you are recovering from an injury, or if you have limited mobility. It's a good addition to a cross-training program, because yoga works muscles you don't otherwise use. Note that if you have uncontrolled high blood pressure or retinopathy, you should not place your head below your waist.

Another gentle form of exercise that anyone can do that increases flexibility, along with balance, is T'ai Chi (Taijiquan). You learn a series of slow, graceful movements, each one leading to the next. The movements are precise and formal, and it is best to learn T'ai Chi from a teacher, but a video may be a good introduction. Developed as a martial art, millions of people in the Orient use it daily as a combination exercise and meditation. Teachers and students state the benefits as improved concentration, reduced stress, self-confidence, and inner peace.

TRAINING WITH MACHINES

There are machines designed to give you a cardiovascular workout, and there are machines designed to increase your muscle strength and tone. If you join an athletic club or gym or participate in a medically supervised program, you'll have the opportunity to exercise on some state-of-the-art equipment. Try not to be intimidated by their complex appearance. You may be happily surprised by the benefits they'll bring to your exercise routine. You may be able to ride further on a stationary bike than a real one. You can burn the same amount of calories on a stairclimber, and with less body impact, than you would while jogging. And when weather is at its extremes, you'll want to exercise indoors.

Choosing home exercise equipment.

Buying an exercise machine for your home use may sound like a great idea: it's convenient, private, and always available, plus you can chat with your family or watch your favorite television shows while you exercise. If it's such a great idea, why are the want ads full of home exercise machines for sale?

This is for several reasons. First, when you exercise at home, you don't get the supervision you need if you have problems or questions. You may find yourself in a holding pattern, with no idea how to progress.

Working out under the direction of trainers at an athletic club or medically supervised program helps keep your motivation up. Another reason is that exercise machines that are *1*) fun to use, *2*) don't break down all the time, *3*) give you information to keep you motivated (calories burned, miles traveled), and *4*) high quality are very expensive. So, most people buy less expensive ones that break down often, are boring, or don't give a high-quality aerobic workout. Yet another reason is that people change their minds about how they want to spend their time exercising. They may get tired of rowing or prefer to bike outside.

The point is that before you spend $100 or $3,000 on a home exercise machine, make sure you really will use it. Decide where you're going to put it. If you have to store it away in a closet, you might be less likely to use it. Shop around as much as you can. Try the equipment out before buying by putting it through a typical exercise session. Shopping will be much easier if you're already used to working out on exercise machines at a gym or athletic club. Make sure the equipment has some sort of warranty and be clear on the limits of that warranty. Machines need service, so expect to spend money on having someone come to your home to take care of it.

Stationary bicycles.

Riding a stationary bicycle not only gives you a great aerobic workout, but it can help strengthen your legs and build muscular endurance. Biking is a non-weight-bearing activity. This means that the bike carries your weight. Along with your cardiovascular system, your legs and hips get the most benefit from a workout on a stationary bike.

Stationary bikes come in two basic models: upright and recumbent. The difference lies in how your body weight is distributed on the bike. An upright bike places your body weight down your spine to between your legs. You should sit up straight while riding. A recumbent bike allows you to pedal while leaning back rather than sitting straight up. Your buttocks support your weight, and this position may be more comfortable for you than having the bike saddle between your legs. Because this position allows you to recline somewhat, there is the possiblity of increased overall blood circulation compared with an upright bike. Both upright and recumbent bikes provide a hearty, safe workout.

Adjust the seat position so that your leg is never completely straight while pedalling. There should be a slight bend at your knee when your leg is extended.

The more expensive stationary bikes have different programs so you can vary your workout. The "hill" program will warm you up, then let you ride over a series of increasingly difficult hills, then cool you down. It does this by varying the resistance against which you're pedaling. A "steady" program will keep your resistance at the same level throughout your workout. A "random" program will vary the resistance randomly every so often. With the last two programs, you should warm up before you start biking. The expensive bikes will also keep track of your time, mileage, and calories burned.

If you're thinking of buying home exercise equipment, a good stationary bike may be the right choice. Exercise bicycles are generally the least expensive of all exercise equipment. Look for sturdy construction—make sure it will support your weight. Figure out how the bike gives you the resistance you're pedaling against.

Some bikes add resistance with a brake pad applied to the wheel, much like the brake on a typical 10-speed bike; avoid these. Some stationary bikes have a belt that is cinched around a flywheel. The tighter the belt is cinched on the flywheel, the more resistance you get as you pedal. Avoid a bike that has a soft rubber flywheel because the rubber can change shape when you apply the tension, giving you a jerky motion as you pedal. Choose one made of metal instead. The other type of resistance is created by turning a fan. Machines that allow you to pedal while alternately pumping handles with your arms will give you the extra advantage of working the upper and lower body at the same time. This is similar to cross-country skiing machines, except that the exercise is non–weight bearing.

Check the bike for fit. Make sure the handle bars raise high enough so that your knees won't hit them. Can you adjust the seat height? Does it stay put once you've adjusted it? You'll appreciate a well-fitted, well-padded seat after a few minutes of cycling.

Treadmills.

A treadmill allows you to walk or run in place without having to go outside. You can read or watch television and still cover a few miles each day. You get your workout by adjusting two things: how fast the rubber walking area is moving and how hard you have to work. Work intensity can be increased by simulated uphill walking. Expensive treadmills can lift their front ends off the ground, so that you're walking uphill. The greater the angle, the harder you have to work. Expensive treadmills also have programs that warm you up and cool you down after the main part of your workout. You'll be able to track your mileage, time, and calories burned.

A heavy-duty treadmill can be expensive—$3,000 or more, although you can find one that's good for a walking program for $800 to $1,000. Treadmills are more prone to break down than other exercise equipment. You'll want to make sure a good warranty is included. Some companies offer a service contract for an additional fee, which could be a wise investment.

When buying a treadmill, look for one with stable footing. Make sure your feet don't slip easily. Choose one with side rails or bars that you can grab onto in case you do slip. Make sure the controls are easy to reach so that you can adjust the speed and stop it quickly when exercising.

Stairclimbers.

These machines simulate walking up stairs and can offer either a strenuous or light aerobic workout. They're not for everyone. The advantage is that, although stairclimbers can provide a hard workout, they are easy on the legs and joints because little impact is placed on the body. But if your posture is wrong as you exercise, you won't get the maximum workout. It's important to stand straight up. Use the handrails for balance only; don't lean on them.

It's important to warm up thoroughly before you begin to climb. Start climbing at a low intensity, or consider a 10-minute warm up on a stationary bike first. Your first few stairclimbing sessions should be limited to 5 minutes or less at the lowest intensity until you're sure it's a good exercise for you. Ask for training on how to use the machine before you start. The machines will measure your time, number of flights climbed, and calories burned.

Many stairclimbers offer resistance through

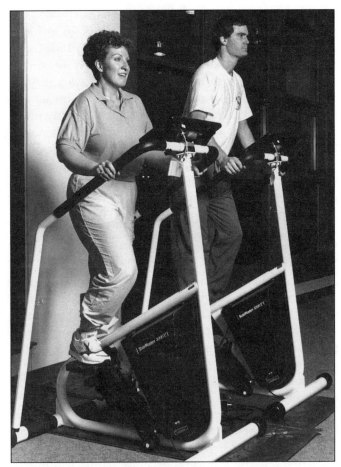

Good posture will help you get the best workout on a stairclimbing machine.
Photograph by Les Todd, courtesy of Duke University Photo Department.

hydraulics much like the shocks on your car. Most of the work is through leg power and the force of your weight. Your movements should be fluid and comfort-able. Some machines have electric motors to control the speed and smooth the movement.

If you're considering buying a stairclimber, avoid the inexpensive ones, especially ones without handrails. The movement should be smooth and fluid, and you should be able to vary the resistance. Avoid machines that jar you when your down foot hits the lowest point.

Rowing machines.

These can give you a great aerobic workout plus help strengthen your legs, arms, back, shoulders, and abdomen. But you have to be sure you use the proper technique. Poor technique can lead to injuries—partic-ularly to the back. If you've had a back injury or problems, check with your doctor before working out on a rowing machine.

When you row, it is important to keep your back straight. You should push with your legs and gradually bring your arms in. You shouldn't push off with your arms and back. If you feel any back strain or pain, ask for training on proper technique. Instruction should include proper breathing technique, too.

There are different types of rowing machines. One type uses pistons that look like shock absorbers. The pistons are attached to the oars—so that the resistance is placed on the oars. However, you may not be able to adjust the resistance on this type of machine, which makes it difficult for you to progress once you get in better shape.

Another type is a flywheel rower. This type best simulates actual rowing because the flywheel keeps spinning even when you stop rowing. This allows you to pick up momentum as you row. By adjusting the gearing of the wheel or opening or closing the wind damper, you can change the resistance. The faster the blades spin, the more resistance you will feel.

If you're thinking of buying a rowing machine, look for one that has a sturdy construction. Make sure the frame doesn't bow when you sit on it. It should be heavy enough so that it doesn't move or jump along the room as you row. The seat should glide evenly on the track while supporting your weight. Check the fit. Can you extend your legs fully when you stroke? Do you have to lean too far to reach the handles? Leaning too far can put a strain on your back.

Cross-country skiing machines.

Cross-country skiing machines will give you an aerobic workout plus help you develop your upper and lower body because the machine places resistance on both your legs and your arms to simulate real skiing. The weight-bearing exercise is good for your overall fitness. Most machines have electronic speedometers that will show the time and distance of and calories burned in your workout.

If you want to buy a cross-country skiing machine, be sure you really enjoy this type of exercise first. This exercise requires skill. Make sure you're committed to using it before you spend the money. Work out on one at a gym or athletic club for a few weeks. When shopping, check that the skis glide smoothly. They shouldn't grab or stick as you move on them. The height and the resistance of the arm poles or ropes should be adjustable. And the skis should have toe straps to keep your feet in place as you exercise.

Your VCR.

One of the least expensive exercise machines is your videotape player. Consider exercising with an aerobic dance videotape. These tapes can give you the feel of participating in an aerobics class. They can help you get a good workout, and if you feel uncomfortable about exercising in front of others, these are a good alternative to an aerobics class. The disadvantage is that you won't have an instructor to correct your form and supervise your workout. For these reasons, exercise videos are safer if you're a veteran of aerobics classes.

Before you purchase a tape, rent one to see if you like it. You'll also have to consider the following:

- Safety. Make sure that the floor in your home offers good support and cushion. Don't exercise on a concrete floor. You want a floor that has some give to it. You're better off not exercising on deep carpet that will inhibit you from moving your feet from side to side easily. It really helps to work out in front of a mirror so you can compare your form to that shown on the tape.
- Room to move around. If you don't have adequate space in your home (in the room where the television is) then working out with a videotape won't be a good option. You don't want to crash into a chair or swing your arm into a lamp.
- While trying out new tapes, look for safety tips before and during the routine and whether it offers good instruction on how to do each routine. The good tapes often offer lower-level exercises for those who are just starting out.
- Consider buying more than one tape. After some time, you'll likely get bored with the same tape and routines. If you have two or three, you can alternate them.

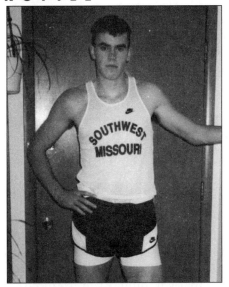

than just find a sport he liked—he broke his high school record for 1,600 meters with a time of 4:17:3. He was also All-State in the half mile and in cross-country.

What is it that appeals to Tom about running track? In a word: discipline. Of running with diabetes, Tom says, "I never let it stop me from doing anything." Tom's high school teammates and coach knew about his diabetes. They were curious, and he explained about taking insulin and what insulin does. For the most part he says, people have been supportive.

The summer before beginning his freshman year at Southwest Missouri State, Tom developed his own workout schedule, which included a 6- to 8-mile morning run followed by running stadium

steps. In the afternoon, he would jump rope and do sit-ups and push-ups. Some days, he also took an evening run of about 4 miles. When he's running, Tom carries two glucose tablets with him, so he is prepared if his blood glucose level should go too low. But he says reactions have not been a problem.

Tom checks his blood glucose four times a day and tests after he runs. His current running goal? Lowering his time for the mile. Tom Torbett is one resident of the Show-Me state who can let his track record speak for itself. ∎

"I NEVER LET IT STOP ME FROM DOING ANYTHING."

Talk to Tom Torbett about running track and you quickly get the idea that he'd much rather be out there putting in some miles than talking about it. A freshman at Southwest Missouri State in Springfield, Missouri, Tom started running track in high school. Diagnosed with insulin-dependent diabetes at age two and a half, Tom says he'd always run to keep his blood glucose levels down, but he'd never heard of cross-country until high school. "After a while I started liking it more and more," says Tom with typical modesty. Competing in 800-, 1,600-, and 3,200-meter events, Tom did more

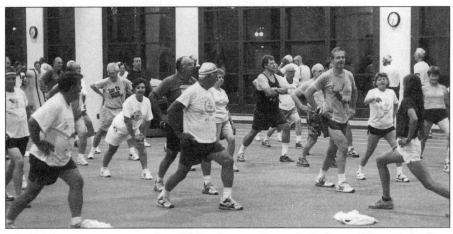

Good aerobics classes always include cool-down stretches.
Photography by Les Todd, courtesy of Duke University Photo Department.

WHERE SHOULD I EXERCISE?

Where you choose to exercise can make all the difference in your results. Part of the exercise experience is enjoying your surroundings. Plenty of people walk not only for fitness but also because their route includes some interesting or relaxing sites. Others stick with an exercise program because they belong to an athletic club that provides trained supervisors and perhaps a dip in the whirlpool for a postworkout reward.

The truth is that, depending on the type of exercise you choose, you can exercise just about anywhere (unless you need to be medically supervised). You just need to decide what you want to do and where you want to do it. Your decision should be based on, among other things, personal tastes, medical needs, time constraints, and financial resources.

Medically supervised programs.

If your diabetes is complicated by cardiovascular disease or if you've had a heart attack, coronary bypass surgery, or trouble with diabetes complications, you may be familiar with medically supervised exercise programs. For people who need specialized care before they begin exercising, these programs are ideal.

If there is a university in your area, they might have a wellness program for health assessment and exercise prescription. Many health-care delivery systems have their own wellness programs or arrangements with other programs. Your doctor may be able to give you a referral. Medically supervised programs offer not only comprehensive health and fitness evaluations, but lifestyle counseling, including diabetes management, nutrition, and behavior modification.

Some larger programs include stays at their facilities for weeks or months while new healthy lifestyle habits are learned. Their staff typically consists of doctors with specialties in cardiology and endocrinology, dietitians, exercise physiologists, educators, and psychologists. These tend to be expensive, although your health insurance may cover some of the expense.

Gyms/athletic clubs.

Gyms and athletic clubs, such as the YMCA or YWCA, have been around for a long time, but they've never been more popular. Some people join them for the social scene; they like to meet people. Some join for the instruction on how to increase fitness. Some join because they want to participate in aerobics classes. Others join for the advanced equipment—many gyms and athletic clubs have an array of exercise equipment that most of us could never afford or have room for in our homes. Some join thinking that the investment will keep them motivated to work out.

Gyms come in all shapes and sizes. Some focus mainly on weight lifting and provide a variety of weight-lifting equipment. Others offer aerobics and yoga classes only. Others emphasize both aerobics and weight training. Some have swimming pools and indoor running tracks. Others include whirlpools, saunas, steam rooms, massage services, and tanning beds. Some have well-trained staff who provide personal training.

One benefit of working out in a gym is the camaraderie of others who are working out. Exercising in an environment where everyone is exercising can be motivating. But some people, particularly those who are just starting out and are out of shape, might be intimidated by exercising in front of people who are in better shape than they are. If you're one of those people, you have nothing to fear. In their advertisements, gyms and athletic clubs may show pictures of beautiful people with big muscles and slender bodies to give you a picture of what you can become, but inside the gym, in addition to the people with the perfect bodies, you'll find people in the same shape as you. And remember, many of those with the beautiful bodies started out much like you and understand what you're going through to get into shape.

Joining can be expensive, and as with any investment, it's wise to carefully think over your goals and your resources and to scout out a facility that will meet your needs before you agree to a long-term membership. Here are some questions your search should answer:

- Will you have a fitness assessment followed by an exercise prescription?
- Does the gym have qualified instructors and fitness experts? Several groups train and certify fitness instructors. The American College of Sports Medicine certifies exercise (aerobics) leaders, health fitness instructors, and specialists in rehabilitation from problems such as heart attack. The American Council on Exercise certifies personal trainers and aerobics instructors. The National Strength and Conditioning Association certifies strength and conditioning specialists. The Aerobic and Fitness Association of America certifies aerobics instructors. The YMCA has an instructor training program; specialists are trained in areas such as rehabilitation from cardiac and back problems through exercise. Find out what your instructors know about diabetes.
- Can you have a trial or daily membership while you decide?
- Are the location and class schedule convenient?
- Are there long lines of people waiting to use the exercise machines? Are the classes always full? Waiting around too long to use an exercise machine or to get into an aerobics class can ruin your enthusiasm and waste your time. On the other hand, a crowded gym can reassure you that the gym is more likely to stay in business.
- Is it financially solvent or likely to disappear overnight, taking your membership with it? Is it part of a chain? Can you work out at "sister" clubs when you travel?

Home workouts.

Here are some good reasons for creating a space in your home to exercise:

- You are reserved or shy and don't like exercising in front of others.
- You are pressed for time, and working out at home can save you the trouble of having to travel somewhere to exercise.
- Your neighborhood isn't safe at times, like the evening, when you want to exercise.
- You don't have the extra money to join a gym or athletic club or you can't find one that's convenient.

Tune into an exercise program on television at the same time each day. Save money for a good exercise machine. Rent exercise videotapes for your VCR.

If you can, exercise in your neighborhood. Plot several walking or biking paths and measure the distances with your car odometer. Vary your paths and patterns for variety and safety.

You can exercise by making everyday projects into a workout. Turn a shopping trip into a brisk walk. Clear out that overgrown area in your yard. Take on that long-overdue painting project or clean out some closets. ❧

CHAPTER 7

Never, never, never quit.
—Winston Churchill

Exercising to *Lose Weight*

YOU'VE DECIDED IT'S TIME TO SHED THOSE UNWANTED POUNDS. That's great! You'll not only look and feel better, but if you have type II diabetes, you'll increase your blood glucose control. If you have type I diabetes, weighing less can mean needing to inject less total insulin. Because having either type of diabetes puts you at risk for additional health problems such as hypertension, high cholesterol, and heart disease, maintaining a healthy, desirable body weight is part of your diabetes control plan.

HOW EXERCISE HELPS YOU LOSE WEIGHT

Coupled with moderate reductions in food, regular exercise is the most effective way to lose weight. In general, if you eat and drink only as many calories as your body needs, your weight will remain about the same. It's when you eat more calories than your body needs that you begin to put on extra weight. Exercise increases your body's need for calories.

Exercise helps you lose weight by burning off calories. In addition, exercise increases the rate at which your body burns calories even when you aren't exercising (called your resting metabolic rate). This is because exercise builds up your muscle mass as it reduces the amount of body fat. And muscle cells use more energy than fat cells. This means that the effects of exercise can help you burn calories even as you go through your regular daily routine. You may not notice the increase in the rate at which you're burning calories during the day, but you will notice how much better your clothes fit.

Even though exercise uses up lots of calories, you'll get the best results when you combine exercise with a sensible diet. It takes a lot of exercise to burn enough calories to make a difference. To lose one pound of body fat, the average person must use up about 3,500 calories. An average-sized adult has to walk or run six miles or swim for an hour to burn about 500 calories (the equivalent of a fast food hamburger with cheese). You'd have to do this every day for a week to lose just one pound of body weight (real body weight, not just water) through exercise alone. For most of us, exercising this way is unrealistic.

Let's look at an alternative: 30 to 45 minutes of walking, four times a week, will use up about 210 to 280 calories during each walk. If you also decrease your calorie intake by 500 calories on five days that week, you've eliminated 3,500 calories. You've just lost a pound in a healthy, sensible way.

The bottom line is that you need to combine exercise with moderate adjustments in your diet if you want to lose weight and keep it off. One without the other isn't as effective as the two combined. You'll notice the results faster, too. But remember, if you really want permanent weight loss, you've got to make permanent changes in your lifestyle.

THE LINK BETWEEN DIABETES AND BODY WEIGHT

Type II diabetes and being overweight are connected. Somehow, carrying excess body fat increases your body's resistance to the action of insulin. If you have type II diabetes, you may be taking glucose-lowering drugs such as an oral sulfonylurea or injected insulin to help overcome insulin resistance. Losing weight can mean no longer needing these medications.

If you have type I diabetes and are overweight, you need to inject more insulin than you would if you were at your healthy body weight. This is for the same reason as for people with type II diabetes—to overcome insulin resistance. This is not only expensive, but it can lead to gaining even more weight. Here's the connection: If you have extra insulin available in your body, it will do what it does best, which is take glucose from the blood and store it in body cells. This may also make you feel hungrier, so you may eat more than normal, leading to more weight gain. If you want to lose weight, it's important to match the amount of insulin closely to your needs through self-monitoring of blood glucose.

Closely matching insulin to body needs leads many people to try intensive insulin therapy. The aim of this therapy is to keep blood glucose levels as close to normal as possible, through multiple (three or more) daily insulin injections and blood glucose checks. Near-normal blood glucose control effectively prevents the onset and worsening of diabetes complications of the eyes, kidneys, and nerves, but there are two unpleasant side effects: hypoglycemia and weight gain.

Hypoglycemia occurs because you are injecting insulin more often in order to keep blood glucose levels in the normal range (under 120 mg/dl except during the first hour or two after a meal). You no longer have a blood glucose "cushion" when you eat a little less food or have a little more excitement or exercise. So it doesn't take much to have a hypoglycemic reaction.

What causes the weight gain? Intensive insulin therapy allows your body to use the energy you take in as food more efficiently. There is much less glucose leaving your body in urine, so every calorie you take in counts. Stopping this calorie loss through urine accounts for most of the weight gain. If you are already in fairly good control, you don't normally lose as many calories this way as someone in poorer control, so your weight gain will probably be less. The other part to this weight gain is that overall metabolic rate decreases. Probably for many reasons, not yet understood, tight control helps your metabolism become more efficient. That is, it does the same amount of "work" keeping your body functioning, but uses less calories to do it. Part of this may be because your body spends less energy breaking down fat stores when insulin is in short supply and then rebuilding fat stores when insulin is available. This futile cycling of fat becomes less common with intensive insulin therapy.

Your need for regular exercise increases with intensive insulin therapy. Along with a low-fat diet, exercise will allow you to avoid or drop those extra pounds. Exercise makes you more sensitive to insulin, and you need less total insulin for the same level of blood glucose control. Using less insulin may help you control your appetite. If you plan to begin intensive insulin therapy, a slight decrease in daily calorie intake, especially fat, and an increase in your regular exercise routine should prevent weight gain.

EXERCISE FOR BEGINNERS

If you've lived a sedentary life, thinking of starting an exercise program may be hard. But then again, the fact that you're reading this book indicates that it's at least something you're considering. Eliminate your excuses for not starting and begin today.

A common mistake is trying to do too much, too soon. You could get discouraged or injure yourself. You'll guarantee success if you set realistic goals, begin slowly, and gradually increase the amount you do. The more times you exercise, the better you'll get at it, and you'll begin to really enjoy it! It takes most people several months of practice before exercise becomes a habit.

A good start is to think about some simple ways you can begin increasing your level of activity in your everyday life. For example, walk more and take the car less. Take the first spot you see in a parking lot, far from the store door, and walk. Get off the bus a few stops earlier and walk the rest of the way. Bike to a friend's house instead of driving. Take the stairs instead of an elevator.

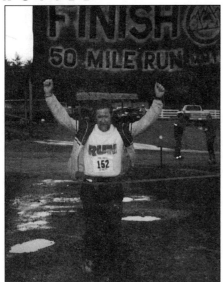

"I REACHED A POINT WHERE I WAS RUNNING FREER."

"I don't know that there was ever a real time in my life that I did exercise. I guess I was a fairly active teenager, but I was never involved in anything like a structured exercise program. Over the years I picked up weight. I picked up quite a bit of weight. I would go on diets and lose the weight. I was going up and down, up and down. By the time I was diagnosed with diabetes, I was physically in very poor shape. I could not walk up a flight of stairs without getting totally out of breath." Leland Gammon's words probably have a familiar ring to many people with type II diabetes.

Leland, a resident of Lynchburg, Virginia, was 38 when he was diagnosed with diabetes. Although the news caught him off guard, he'd known that something was seriously wrong. During a three-week period before he was diagnosed, he lost close to 30 pounds. His big fear: heart trouble. But instead the diagnosis was diabetes.

Leland's physician explained that exercise was an important component of diabetes care along with diet and medication. "But he let me have the freedom to pick the exercise I wanted. I knew it would have to be an individual sport such as biking or running." He had volunteered at the Virginia 10-Miler, a nationally renowned footrace, for several years. Running seemed like an appealing possibility.

But Leland recalls he had to walk before he could run. He spent a week in the hospital after diagnosis, learning about diabetes management, how to inject insulin, and how to establish a healthy diet for life. Once his blood glucose level was stabilized with insulin, his first goal was to take off some more weight. "In the beginning, all I did was walk, and I lost weight," he says. "I can't remember my exact weight when I began walking, but I know neither my doctor nor I wanted me to run until I was under 200 pounds." Once below 200 pounds, Leland was able to go off medication and to control his diabetes with diet and exercise. He began a cautious running program. "It actually took me three months of running to run one mile without stopping. When I first started, I gasped for air, and my legs burned. Then, all of a sudden, I reached a point where I was running freer, easier, and more comfortably." Despite stabilizing his weight and staying with an exercise program, Leland has subsequently had to resume insulin therapy to control his diabetes.

Although Leland's approach to exercise is cautious, he's racked up some remarkable accomplishments. After running for several years and completing six marathons, Leland set his sights on running an ultramarathon. In 1990, after seven months of careful training, he ran the Mountain Masochist 50-Mile Trail Run, completing the race within the 12-hour time limit.

One fringe benefit of his exercise conversion: his wife Peggy also took up running. Now, Leland and Peggy run together several evenings during the week and on weekends. Leland says running together has given the couple special time together and brought a new closeness to their 30-year marriage.

In celebration of their 30th wedding anniversary, Leland and Peggy planned a hiking vacation in Arizona. With characteristic care, Leland plotted his training routine, adding some weight training and stairclimbing workouts to be ready for their rigorous hikes. "I always take everything slow," says Leland. "I listen to my body. I approach things in a real common sense way."

Today, Leland's exercise routine includes five-mile runs three nights a week, with longer runs on Saturday and Sunday. Ten years after being diagnosed with diabetes Leland says, "I always felt like being diagnosed with diabetes was a blessing. I needed something and I needed it about the time it happened. It saved my life. I have a totally different outlook on life, and I'm much happier. I enjoy life now. It's because of the lifestyle changes that came about as a result of being diagnosed with diabetes." ■

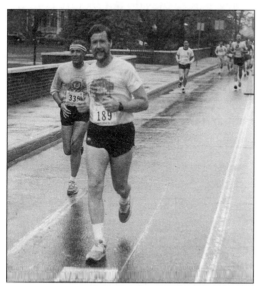

Diabetes therapy, Leland style.

Get up during television commercials and do some housework. Take a brisk walk during your lunch hour instead of overeating. Every extra effort you make will be rewarded by adding to your fitness.

At the same time, you might be ready to begin a regular exercise program. The best way to work off unwanted pounds is through regular aerobic exercise. Aerobic exercise is continuous, meaning that you perform it for some time (such as 15, 20, or more minutes after warming up) without stopping. Aerobic exercise raises your heart rate and prompts your body to use more oxygen. Over time, it leads to cardiovascular fitness—healthy heart, blood vessels, and lungs.

Examples of aerobic exercise include walking, bicycling, swimming, aerobic dance, cross-country skiing, running, and jogging. You also can have an aerobic

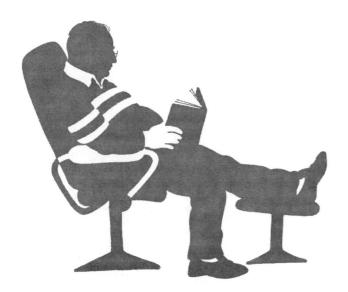

workout on a treadmill, stationary bike, rowing machine, and stairclimbing machine. Any of these will help you achieve a high level of physical fitness and help you lose weight.

If you are very overweight, have problems or pain in your joints and ligaments (such as arthritis), or are unable to move freely, good choices for aerobic exercise are exercising in a pool or while sitting in a chair. The water or the chair will support your weight so that it doesn't bear down on your joints or legs and feet. You can still get a great aerobic workout—you just need to know some exercises to try. See the Chapter 8 for examples of these types of exercises. Ask members of your health-care team for their recommendations.

Sports such as football, baseball, and golf are not considered aerobic because they do not require continuous movement. When you play these sports, you start and expend energy quickly but in small amounts, stop, and start again. (Remember: if you get to stand still for very long, it's not aerobic.) If you enjoy playing these sports, don't despair: most provide a good total-body workout, and you will still benefit by participating in them. Consider doing them on the two or three days that you don't do aerobic exercise.

If you've been inactive for quite a while and are more than just a little overweight, even walking around the block may present a challenge. You'll need to gradually build up to a comfortable workout level. You might want to begin by doing a few gentle stretches and then walking for 5 or 10 minutes at "conversational" intensity (you are able to carry on a conversation, but not able to sing), then stop and rest a few minutes, and then repeat the walk for another 5 or 10 minutes. Cool down by walking slower for a few minutes and repeating the gentle stretches. Every week, add 3 to 5 minutes to your total walking time. Eventually, you'll be able to complete an entire 30- to 45-minute workout without resting.

To lose weight, you should focus on how long you exercise and not on how hard you exercise. It is better for you to exercise for 20 or 30 minutes at a mild-to-moderate pace without stopping than to use up all your energy working very hard for 10 or 15 minutes.

AEROBICS AND WEIGHT LOSS

The bottom line is that aerobic exercise is great for losing weight. Because you keep exercising for an extended period, aerobic exercise burns the most calories. Don't think you have to push yourself to the limit when you do aerobic exercise. The common-sense guideline is: if you feel like you're working too hard, you probably are. If you've had exercise testing and an exercise prescription, you'll know how hard to work. If not, you need to know whether the pace you're using is safe for you. Get your doctor's okay, especially if you used a heart rate formula to find your target workout heart rate (see Chapter 4).

It's true that some exercises burn more calories faster than others because they require you to work harder in a shorter period of time. But don't choose an exercise solely by how many calories you can burn. Exercise is work, but it doesn't have to be drudgery. It's more fun when you choose exercises that you enjoy and will continue doing. The key to permanent weight loss is regular exercise and moderate eating. You don't want to take the crash diet approach and wait to start exercising until you've lost a little weight. Make exercise a regular part of your life each day, just like sleeping and eating.

BUT EXERCISE MAKES ME HUNGRY!

You've probably heard someone say that, although they want to lose weight, they'd rather use diet alone, because exercise makes them so hungry that they eat too much. It is true that if you exercise very hard for an hour or more that you'll probably need to eat afterward. Your stomach could even be growling. But for most of us, this type of exercise is not in our plans.

If your workout is low-intensity aerobic exercise, just enough to reach and maintain your target heart rate for 20 to 45 minutes, exercise may actually decrease your desire for food. In fact, if you are supposed to eat dinner afterward, you may want less food than normal. Some researchers believe that this happens because exercise promotes the release of hormones that decrease appetite.

If your stomach is growling and you feel hungry, it means you need some food. Go ahead and have a snack or, if it's mealtime, eat your meal. Eating something to keep your stomach from growling after you exercise will not cancel out your efforts. The benefits of exercise far outweigh the "damage" that some extra calories can do. Be aware, however, if you start to use a little exercise as an excuse to eat a lot more, even when you're not hungry.

THE MYTHS ABOUT DIETING

Why can't you just go on a strict diet, lose some weight, and skip the exercise? Because most diets don't work alone if you want to achieve permanent weight loss. Exercise helps you maintain your weight loss.

A diet that severely restricts calories is dangerous for anyone, especially for those of us with diabetes. Rapid weight loss can cause dehydration, nausea, dizziness, and impaired kidney function. It can also result in loss of muscle tissue, which lowers metabolic rate. If you inject insulin, such a diet could cause severe swings in blood glucose levels.

You probably know people (maybe even yourself) who have gone on a diet, lost ten pounds, and within a short time gained it all back (and sometimes more). Why is this? Did they eat more after their diets to make up for lost time? Possibly. Maybe they thought that once they'd lost that weight, they could splurge a little (or a lot) more often. Returning to old unhealthy eating habits guarantees you'll return to the old unhealthy weight.

The real problem behind diets is that over time your body responds to the diet in a way that is contrary to what you're trying to achieve. Let's say you decide to go on a low-calorie diet. You do without a substantial part of the food you normally eat. After a few days, you step on the scale and discover that you've lost five pounds. That's real progress, right? Wrong.

While you were depriving yourself of food, your body went on the defensive. For starters, when you began your diet, your body first began to use the carbohydrate stored in your body as glyco-gen for fuel and in the process lost a lot of water. This loss registered on your bathroom scale. But your body doesn't like to be dehydrated. Soon you'll make up the deficit by replacing the fluid you lost and rapidly gain back many of those pounds you so proudly shed.

Another interesting thing happens when you go on a diet. When you lose weight rapidly, you also lose protein from muscles and organs, minerals, and bone, together known as lean (or fat-free) body mass. Nearly 25 percent of the weight you lose by dieting and not exercising will be from lean body mass. You don't want to lose muscle. Exercise helps preserve muscle mass while you diet. Muscle is a valuable resource for burning calories because it takes a lot more energy for your body to maintain muscle than it does fat.

Muscles contain protein. Protein is made up of amino acids. Some amino acids constantly pass from the muscles to the bloodstream and back to the muscles again. It takes energy to go through this process. Although the more active a tissue is, the more energy it needs to maintain itself, even at rest your muscles are burning calories.

Muscles burn more calories than fat. Fat, on the other hand, requires far less maintenance and contributes little in terms of calories burned. That's why someone who has well-developed muscles burns more calories than someone who weighs the same but who has much more body fat.

Dieting without exercising also lowers your metabolic rate (the rate at which your body burns calories). When you go on a diet, your body recognizes that it isn't getting as much food as it once did. In defense, it tries to decrease energy output. This makes it more difficult to continue to lose weight and keep it off.

MAKING CHANGES IN YOUR DIET

Very-low-calorie diets aren't the answer to permanent weight loss but eating sensibly is. If you're like most people, your biggest battle will be keeping the amount of calories, particularly fat, that you eat down to a reasonable and healthy level so that you can lose weight and keep it off.

To cut out the necessary calories from your diet, it will help to understand the source of your calories. Calories come from four food sources—fats, carbohydrates, protein, and alcohol. Vitamins and minerals do not supply your body with calories, but you need them to release energy from carbohydrates, protein, and fat.

The trick to losing weight is not only cutting down on the amount of calories you eat each day but also decreasing the amount of calories you get from fat. Compare the amount of calories that are in one gram of fat to that in carbohydrates, protein, and alcohol:

- One gram of carbohydrate = 4 calories.
- One gram of protein = 4 calories.
- One gram of fat = 9 calories.
- One gram of alcohol = 7 calories.

As you can see, fat has more than double the number of calories of protein and carbohydrate. Unfortunately, the average American gets almost 40 percent of his or her daily calories from fat (a healthy diet provides less than 30 percent of calories from fat each day). To lose or maintain your weight, you will probably need to cut down on the amount of fat you eat. This means giving up or at least rationing fatty foods such as cookies, chips, ice cream, greasy hamburgers, pepperoni, hot dogs and cold cuts, margarine, butter, full-fat cheeses, and the list goes on.

Get in the habit of reading food labels to see how much fat is contained in the food you eat. Read the food label to find, for each serving of that food, what percentage of calories come from fat. Compare foods and choose the one that is lower in fat.

How much fat can you have in a day? The exact amount of fat to eat each day varies from person to person. A general recommendation is that less than 30 percent of your total daily calories should come from fat. You'll need to count your daily fat intake in two ways: 1) the number of calories in a food that are due to the fat, and 2) the number of grams of fat in a food. The amount of fat in grams that you can eat depends on how many calories you eat each day.

Let's say you eat 1,500 calories each day. To determine the number of those calories that should come from fat, multiply 1,500 by 30 percent (1,500 x 0.30) to get 450. A healthy goal for you is to eat no more than 450 calories worth of fat each day. Lowering your intake of calories from fat to this level may start your weight loss.

Most food labels list the amount of fat per serving in grams. So, you'll need to convert your 450 calories from fat into grams. Divide the number of calories from fat (450 in this example) by 9, because 1 gram of fat provides 9 calories (450/9 = 50). To meet the generally recommended daily fat intake, you can eat 50 grams of fat each day if you consume 1,500 total calories a day. If you're already eating 30 percent of calories from fat, you may need to decrease the percentage of fat in your diet to lose weight. Lower the percentage of calories from fat to 20 or 25 percent (1,500 x 0.25 = 375, 375/9 = 42 grams of fat each day). Consult a dietition to find your goals.

To determine how many calories you should eat each day to *maintain* your weight, choose the category

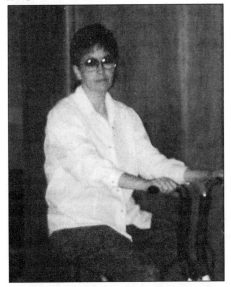

"THERE IS A BETTER WAY OF LIFE." Since the day Pat Pathkiller learned she had diabetes in December 1987, her life has undergone a remarkable transformation. The changes are dramatic: she's down to 155 pounds from an all-time high of 262 pounds. Although bone spurs and legs ulcers once made walking an agony, Pat now rides a stationary bike 10 miles in 36 minutes. But changes like these don't happen overnight. They stem from a commitment to slow, steady progress. In the beginning, Pat recalls, the diagnosis alone was "just about more than I could handle."

Pat's maternal grandmother had had diabetes. She lost both her legs to the disease and her eyesight was failing at the time of her death. When Pat's doctor told her that she, too, had diabetes, Pat says, "I was an emotional wreck. I never had anything hit me so hard in my life, because I saw what my grandmother went through."

But Pat's doctor was encouraging from the start. He felt that if she would eat right and exercise, she would not have to go on insulin. Pat Pathkiller is half Cherokee Indian, and she remains grateful that her doctor did not dismiss her as merely another Native American with diabetes who would wind up on insulin. In fact, Pat says many Native Americans themselves believe that diabetes is inevitable. "You grow up, you get diabetes, and you die. They think that this is what happens to you because you're Native American. I don't want people to feel that way. I want them to know that there is a tomorrow and there is a better way of life," says Pat.

At diagnosis Pat's doctor, sensitive to her emotional turmoil, tried not to overload her with information. He gave her a 1,500-calorie diet sheet and arranged for her to meet with a dietitian in one week. When Pat returned, she was ready to learn. What she found was that she already knew a lot about eating right. She had been on and off diets most

of her life. "I knew what to do, I just needed to be motivated to do it," Pat says.

Pat is very direct about what motivated her: Fear.

How had she let an 100 extra pounds creep onto her 5-foot 9-inch frame so that at age 46, she weighed 262? Pat says, "I had no discipline in my life—where 'I' was concerned. My home was orderly and clean, my husband and my sons were well taken care of—but I was a physical wreck. I had bone spurs in my heels, I had had leg surgeries for ulcers."

Pat's doctor emphasized that exercise would be an important part of keeping her diabetes well controlled. Pat says her initial reaction was "Me? Exercise? I do well to walk!"

After going through what she calls a "pity Pat" phase, Pat did a lot of praying, and with her family's encouragement, she got down to business. Her basic approach was to follow the doctor's orders to the letter.

Pat's husband helped her get going on an exercise routine by presenting her with an exercise bike for their New Year's Eve wedding anniversary (she had been diagnosed right before Christmas). In fact, Pat says the bike now has about 9,700 miles on it and she's ready to trade it in for a new model.

Getting started on exercise was tough Pat says, "because I was so physically unfit I could hardly walk let alone exercise. It's not easy to carry that extra weight around and exercise."

Pat began by riding two miles on the bike and built up from there. As the pounds slowly came off, Pat continued to plug away at her daily bike riding. In the beginning, she did three miles in 30 minutes. Now, five years later, she can ride 10 miles in less than 40 minutes.

She tries to ride every day. If she eats a little extra or feels hungry, she sometimes hops on her bike for a few extra miles. Now that she can walk without pain, Pat incorporates a little walking into her exercise routine when the weather's good.

She's been maintaining her weight loss and healthy lifestyle for more than five years and has never had to go on pills or insulin. Her strategy for handling tempting Native American dishes that spell dietary disaster is simply to avoid them. She's been an inspiration to her community and in 1988 received the Catfish Hunter Hall of Fame Award for her essay on how her life had become healthier since being diagnosed with diabetes.

At 50, Pat's healthier than ever. She credits not only her physician, but especially her family for encouraging her and being willing to make lifestyle changes right along with her. ▪

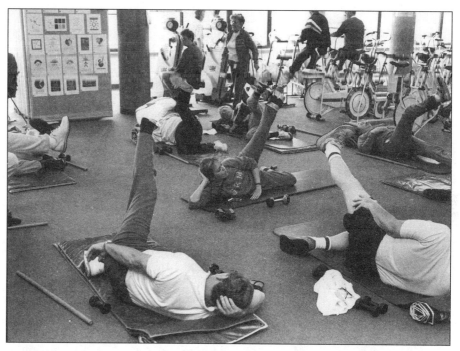

Remember to include strengthening exercises and flexibility stretches in your workout.
Photograph by Les Todd, courtesy of Duke University Photo Department.

below that fits you best. These guidelines are from *Eat for Life* (see Resources).

- If you are not physically active: women, multiply your weight x 3.8 and add 960; men, multiply your weight by 5.5 and add 1080. For example, a couch potato man who weighs 200 pounds requires about 2,180 calories a day (200 x 5.5 = 1,100 + 1080 = 2,180) to maintain that weight.
- If you participate in moderate amounts of activity: women, multiply your weight x 4.5 and add 1120; men, multiply your weight x 6.4 and add 1260.
- If you participate in regular exercise or perform manual labor: women, multiply your weight by 5.1 and add 1280; men, multiply your weight x 7.3 and add 1440.

These are general guidelines for keeping your current weight. You should check with your dietitian, doctor, or another member of your health-care team for precise guidelines to meet your particular needs. But a word of caution: Women should eat no less than 1,200 to 1,500 calories a day, and men should eat no less than 1,500 to 1,800 calories a day. Eating less than these amounts makes it hard to get all the nutrients your body needs to function. Very-low-calorie diets are unhealthy unless you are supervised carefully by your doctor.

If you want to lose one pound of fat in a week, you need to consume about 3,500 calories less than your weekly requirements or 500 calories less a day. The most effective way to do this is to reduce the amount of calories you eat and increase the amount you burn through exercise.

Think of the progress you can make if you eat 500 calories less than your total calories per day. You could lose one pound per week. That's 52 pounds a year! But then consider if you burn an extra 250 calories per day, adding another half pound each week. That is 26 more pounds you could shed and 78 pounds for the whole year. That's 78 pounds you could keep off if you keep up with your exercise and diet routine.

Work with your dietitian, doctor, or diabetes educator to determine the right amount of calories you should eat to meet your needs and to develop a sensible diet plan. Meanwhile, you can begin losing weight by just cutting out one fatty food item each day. If you supplement your breakfast with a piece of toast smeared with butter, skip the butter. If a candy bar makes its appearance every day after lunch, cast it aside, and eat one only on Fridays. You'll be amazed at how much little changes in your eating patterns, such as cutting out one or two sources of fat in your meals each day, can help you lose or maintain weight.

Remember, your diet and exercise plan will be most effective and safe if it's created just for you. If you're committed to success, make the extra effort involved in working with your health-care team to form a beneficial and safe weight-loss program. If you require insulin, adjustments may help you reach your goals or

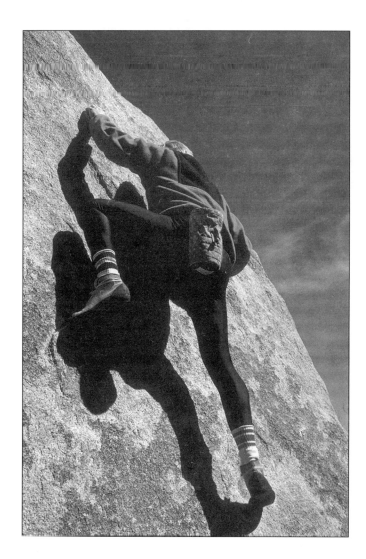

may be needed as you make progress. And it always helps to have more cheerleaders on your sidelines!

STAYING MOTIVATED

One way to keep your exercise routine fun and help keep you motivated is to exercise with a friend. Having a commitment to another fitness-seeker will generally keep you both going. And it's more fun to exercise with someone. When choosing an exercise partner, if you can, find someone who is near the same level of fitness as you are. A person in better physical condition may push you to go beyond what you are capable of doing. Others may hold you back.

Reaching for goals will also keep you in there rolling along. See Chapter 2 for ideas on goal setting.

People who get bored with one particular exercise day after day cross-train. This means alternating between exercises that use different muscle groups. For example, you might walk one day, ride a bike the next, and swim another day. The key is making exercise fun so that you will do it and look forward to it. 🍃

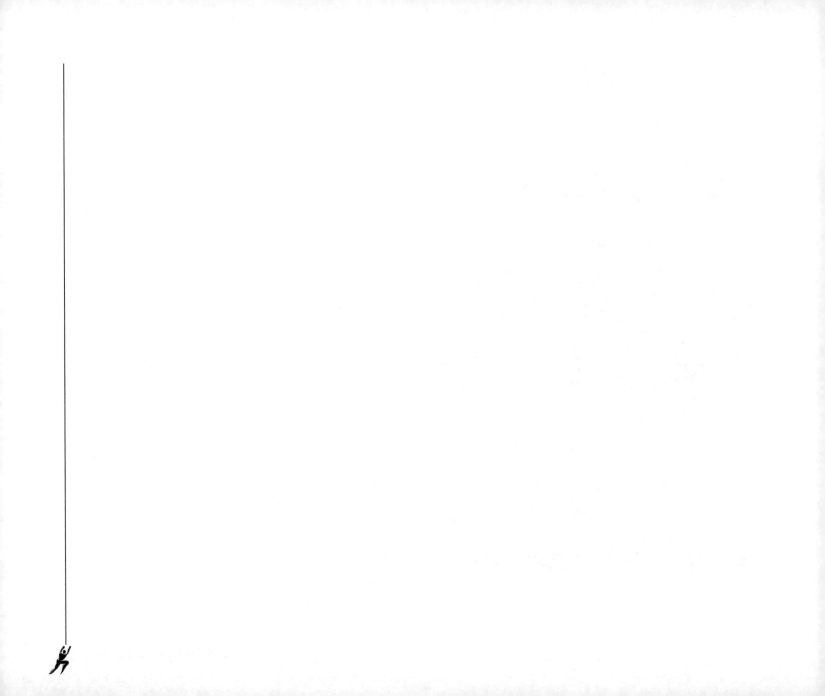

CHAPTER 8

Exercising With *Special* Needs

E XERCISE IS IMPORTANT FOR EVERYONE WITH DIABETES. And almost everyone, regardless of their physical abilities, can exercise. Just because you aren't able or willing to run a marathon doesn't mean you can't have fun and gain the health benefits of exercise. But some people aren't believers. They've convinced themselves that exercise is impossible because they are either too old, too burdened with a physical disability, or too overweight for exercise to make any difference.

Have you heard of the *disuse syndrome*? This is a term used to describe what happens to your body when a particular physical problem like vision, surgery, or some other impairment keeps you from being physically active. When you've been inactive or confined to bed rest, all the systems in the body suffer. Your body as a whole starts to function less effectively, because its parts are not getting the needed stimulation of muscular contraction. Muscles need to be worked. If they aren't being used, they begin to atrophy or deteriorate—sometimes to a point where they won't perform even when you try to do even the easiest task such as taking the garbage out. The disuse syndrome occurs in people of all ages.

The remarkable thing about muscles, however, is that you can increase their efficiency and reverse the disuse syndrome through regular exercise. This is great news to someone who hasn't been as active as he or she once was but wants to turn his or her lifestyle around.

You don't have to train like an Olympian to benefit from exercise. Few people train like that. You will increase your fitness with something as simple as a walk in the neighborhood several times a week, a home exercise program, or a regular swim in the pool. You can find an exercise program perfect for you and your health, and your diabetes control will improve, and you'll feel so much better!

The first step in planning an exercise program is safety. It is important to have a preexercise examination and to receive an exercise prescription before you begin. During this process, your health-care team will identify any exercise limitations you have. They should discuss any possible side effects that medications you take can cause if combined with certain activities. The result will be an exercise program tailored to your individual needs, no matter your age and whether you're obese, pregnant, or hampered by a diabetes complication.

EXERCISE FOR THE OLDER GENERATIONS

As we age, our physical abilities decline. As you've gotten older, you may have noticed that it's a little tougher to do some of the things you used to do quite easily, such as mowing the lawn, washing the car, or performing other household chores. Some of this has to do with getting older. But a lot of it happens to us because we allow ourselves to become more inactive as we get older.

If you haven't been exercising, don't worry. It's never too late to start an exercise program. Exercise should be a regular part of your diabetes management at any age, but not every exercise program is for everyone. There might be some exercise programs that you should avoid because of your particular health condition or certain medications you take.

Exercise can make a world of difference to you as you get older. Sure, your reaction times may be slower, and you might not be able to work out as strenuously as you once did. But many older people who regularly exercise, regardless of their ages, are able to move about and perform physical tasks much more easily than those who don't exercise. For example, people find that after a period of regular exercise they are able to perform household tasks easier and walk farther without getting tired. They have more energy to do things. And they feel a lot better.

You'll need to remember that, as you age, it takes longer to adapt to exercise. Exercises you did years before won't be as easy. Jogging has become walking.

Hitting a tennis ball might require more effort. Even lifting groceries out of the car can be a challenge. You might find that decreased flexibility and strength, arthritis, circulatory problems, and diabetes complications can place some restrictions on the exercises you can do.

Start slowly and gradually increase how hard and how long you exercise. If you work too hard when you're new to an exercise program, your extra efforts might reward you with an injury and put your exercise program on hold while you recover. To increase your opportunity for success, it's important to pick an exercise intensity and frequency (per week) that you can live with. Too many times, people will sabotage their new exercise plan by exercising too often and too hard—so hard that they are sore and reluctant to exercise again.

As you exercise, your heart rate should not rise too quickly or too high. Diabetes and certain medications, such as those used to treat blood pressure, can alter your heart rate and affect your tolerance to exercise. Therefore, don't rely on a standard heart rate formula to determine what your target heart rate should be during exercise. To determine a safe exercising heart rate, you may need to have an exercise stress test. That test will help define the type and intensity of exercise that you can try.

Generally, it is not a good idea to choose exercises that require fast movements and quick changes of direction, because coordination and reaction time slow with age. Seniors should avoid exercises that require straining or holding their breath. Such exercises can cause blood pressure to rise too much, which can place too much stress on the heart and circulatory system.

There are many activities to choose from. The following are a few good choices for people who are older. Discuss these exercises with your health-care team to determine the best options for you. And experiment with different exercises to discover which ones you like best.

Walking.

This is a great way to get fit, and almost anyone can do it. After all, you've been doing it since you were about one year old! If you've been inactive for some time, even 5 minutes of continuous walking might seem like a lot. But if you walk each day, you'll soon be able to walk for 30 minutes at a time or more.

When starting out, try to add about three to five minutes to your walking time each week. By adding duration (the length of time you walk) to your walks instead of intensity (how fast you walk), you can safely progress in your workouts. For the best health benefit, walk at a conversational intensity. In other words, while you walk you should still be able to carry on a conversation. Find a pace that suits you and stick with it for most of your walk. Use a slightly slower pace for your warm up and cool down. A good goal to shoot for is to walk for 30 to 45 minutes, five (or more) days a week. Count on taking several months to reach this goal.

If the weather is severe—either too hot or too cold—don't exercise outside. On such days, take your walking program inside. Many senior citizen groups have organized "mall walks." These groups walk in indoor shopping malls before the shops open in the morning. These walks are a great way to meet other people who have goals similar to yours—they want to stay fit. Check with your local indoor shopping malls, senior centers, or YMCAs to see whether such groups exist in your area. But don't forget that this is one activity you can do on your own anytime the mall doors are open.

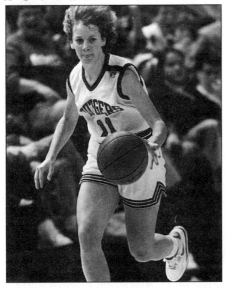

"I'M THE KIND OF PERSON WHO WON'T GIVE UP."

For Cheryl Cop, freshman year of college held the promise of great things to come. A basketball player since age seven, Cheryl was heavily recruited by colleges during her senior year of high school. Choosing Rutgers University wasn't hard. The women's basketball team was highly rated. The New Brunswick campus was near her hometown of Elizabeth, New Jersey. Academically, the school was well regarded. And most important, Rutgers had coach Theresa Grentz.

Playing NCAA Division One women's basketball is the pinnacle for someone who has loved the game since the day her dad nailed up a backyard hoop. Then things started to go wrong.

It began with an injury. In January 1990, Cheryl, who plays point guard, tore the anterior cruciate ligament in her right knee. At first, she tried rehabilitating the knee and playing with a knee brace. When that didn't work, she had knee surgery to repair the ligament in March. After the surgery, Cheryl was on crutches for six weeks. She was losing weight but thought it was from the exertion of walking around on crutches. Finally, she went to see a doctor. She had all the classic symptoms. The diagnosis was type I diabetes.

By the end of freshman year, Cheryl had been hit by a serious injury and diabetes. She responded to the double blow with determination. "When I first hurt my knee, I was kind of doubtful about coming back, but I had talked to a lot of other people who had torn a ligament and come back, so I was optimistic," she says. "When the diabetes hit, I remember my team doctor saying there was no reason why I couldn't play basketball any more."

That summer, Cheryl faced two hurdles: getting her knee back into shape and getting her diabetes under control for elite athletic competition. Looking back, Cheryl says her competitive drive fueled her determination to make it back on the court. "By nature I'm the kind of person who won't give up. I'd been playing basketball since I was seven. I was at least going to give it a shot."

Cheryl's summer was dedicated to rehabilitating her knee and learning to live well with diabetes. Every day she worked at getting her knee back into shape. Warming up her knee first by soaking it in a whirlpool, she'd ride a stationary bike for an hour, lift weights, and then work with a trainer to regain her knee's range of motion. She checked in with her endocrinologist once a week, reporting her blood glucose readings and fine-tuning her insulin dosage. By the end of the summer, she felt the hard work had paid off.

But Cheryl found that diabetes would demand more adjustments. "During the summer months," Cheryl recalls, "I was doing the same thing every day. But once school started it was another change. I had to adjust to my school schedule. I had to make sure I ate my three meals. It was a tough time my first year coming back. Everything was new to me with diabetes." She made it back to play the entire season her sophomore year and has played every year since.

In her senior year, Cheryl was able to realize all the promise her freshman year held. She loved playing point guard. "You have to be very knowledgeable about the game. You are responsible for calling a lot of the plays, keeping the team in sync. You are the liaison between the coach and the players out on the court." Looking back to her last season of collegiate play, she remembers the roar of the crowds, the excitement of the games, and the camaraderie of her teammates.

Cheryl's preseason workout consisted of running, conditioning work, and lifting weights to build strength. Practice began November 1, and exhibition games began late in November.

Games take so much energy, even just to warm up, Cheryl usually tried to start out with a blood glucose level around 200. She tested before every game and usually sipped on cola or chocolate milk during the game. Coach Grentz was very supportive, Cheryl says, as were her teammates.

Although she had to make a transition to the workplace, she's confident she'll remain active in sports. She's adamant about the benefits of team sports. "Playing basketball and staying in school at the same time, you learn how to balance your schedule. Also playing on a team, you learn how to work together with other people and overcome hardships. There are good times and bad times."

Cheryl's no nonsense attitude is reflected in her assessment of the impact diabetes has had on her life. "When I was first diagnosed, I wasn't very happy," she says. "But as I look back on it, I think I'm much healthier now—as far as my eating habits. I think my whole situation has made me a stronger person." ■

Water exercises.

Working out in the pool is gaining in popularity and becoming an ideal choice of exercise for older people and people who are rehabilitating from an injury. It's a great form of exercise for people with arthritis or peripheral neuropathy because it doesn't place any stress on the joints or feet. The resistance of the water provides you with a natural way to increase your strength and stamina and reduce the chance of injury.

One type of exercise routine for the water is aqua aerobics. Aqua aerobics involves doing calisthenic-type exercises in waist-deep water. The good part about these exercises is that you don't have to know how to swim to participate. You may wear a flotation belt and exercise without touching the bottom of the pool. This makes it a good choice for those who need to avoid weight-bearing exercises. Check with the YMCA, health clubs, community colleges, or county or city parks to see if they offer aqua aerobics classes.

Another type of water workout is water walking. Some medically supervised programs have pools equipped with a current, which gives you a resistance to push against while you walk. But just walking in waist-deep water along the bottom of the pool or in the ocean is a good way to exercise. Try to work up to walking in the water for up to 30 minutes. Be sure to protect your feet against the bottom of the pool or ocean with shoes you can wear in the water, like Aquasocks.

Swimming itself is an enjoyable and excellent way to stay fit. If you've been inactive for a while, you'll want to begin slowly and not swim too long or too hard. At first, you might want to use a kick board. You can kick, rather than use your arms. The board will keep your upper body afloat, and you won't have to worry about developing a rhythmic breathing pattern. Rhythmic breathing means coordinating arm strokes and turning your head out of the water to take a breath.

Eventually, you might want to combine arm strokes and rhythmic breathing with kicking your legs. If you find it too difficult to combine rhythmic breathing, try using a mask and snorkel. This will help you concentrate on your kicking and arm movements without having to coordinate turning your head to breathe. If you don't want to put your head under water, try swim strokes such as the backstroke or side stroke. If the water bothers your eyes, try a snug but comfortable pair of swimming goggles.

Swimming can be physically challenging, and you will need to start out slowly. To get in shape, you might need to begin by swimming only a few laps, resting, and repeating with a few more laps. At first, 5 to 8 minutes total swimming time might be enough. By alternating rest with work periods, you should be able to build up to swimming continuously for 20 to 30 minutes or more.

Bicycling.

Another great form of exercise is cycling—either indoors on a stationary bicycle or outdoors on a real one. Both forms will help improve your cardiovascular fitness and muscle strength. Cycling is a great choice for people who have orthopedic (spine, bone, or joint) limitations. If your balance or vision is poor, try cycling on a stationary bike or on the back seat of a tandem bike. See Chapter 6 for more on biking technique.

Chair exercises.

If you have difficulty with balance or standing,

chair exercises can help you improve strength, coordination, and flexibility. In as little as 25 minutes a day, you can perform a good chair exercise routine—while you watch television or listen to the radio.

Begin at a low level and gradually build up to a higher level over weeks of practice. Once the exercises seem easy, increase the number of repetitions (the number of times you do each movement). After a few weeks and when you are able to complete 30 repetitions or more, try doing the exercises using some light weights. For example, take two one-pound soup cans and hold one in each hand as you do some arm circles. You can also buy light weights to use during your workouts. Weights that you can strap to your ankles and wrists are good for developing strength. Some weight sets allow you to add more weight as you get stronger. Follow the sample exercises illustrated (next page) or ask your health-care team for instructions on others.

Resistance training.

Resistance or weight training is a good way to develop your endurance, flexibility, and muscle strength. See Chapter 6 for instructions on resistance training. Seniors can participate in resistance training without suffering any injuries or side effects if you get instruction on how to use weights or large rubber bands.

DIABETES COMPLICATIONS

Nerve disease.

Damage to nerves due to diabetes comes in two basic types. One kind is damage to nerves in areas away from the central nervous system, such as hands, arms, feet, and legs. This is known as peripheral neuropathy. The second kind occurs in nerves that control involuntary processes, such as heart rate and digestion. This is called autonomic neuropathy.

Peripheral neuropathy is nerve damage to the extremities. If you have peripheral neuropathy, you may have pain, tingling, and numbness where the nerve damage is. Exercise will not help cure peripheral neuropathy, but the effects of regular exercise will help maintain strength, flexibility, and circulation to the damaged areas. Combined with controlled blood glucose levels, exercise may help relieve the discomfort of neuropathy, although relief can take weeks or months.

During your preexercise exam, you should have discovered whether peripheral neuropathy makes it hard for you to feel pain in particular muscle groups. If so, you'll need to watch that you don't overstretch those muscles while warming up or while exercising.

If you have been inactive for a long time and have peripheral neuropathy, you might not be as flexible as you once were. If so, full range-of-motion stretching exercises might help. These exercise will help you improve flexibility. You can do these exercises for 15 minutes each day as a warm-up to your other exercises. When doing range-of-motion exercises, you slowly and gently move different body parts around the joints—your wrists, elbows, shoulders, ankles, knees, hips, and trunk—forward, back, up, down, and around as far as each will go without causing pain. For example, shrugging your shoulders and doing "windmills" with your arms will loosen up your shoulders. Holding a scarf in each hand and swirling them up, down, and around to music is a fun way to exercise these areas. Ask your doctor or physical therapist to show you how to properly perform these exercises at home.

If peripheral neuropathy has caused numbness in

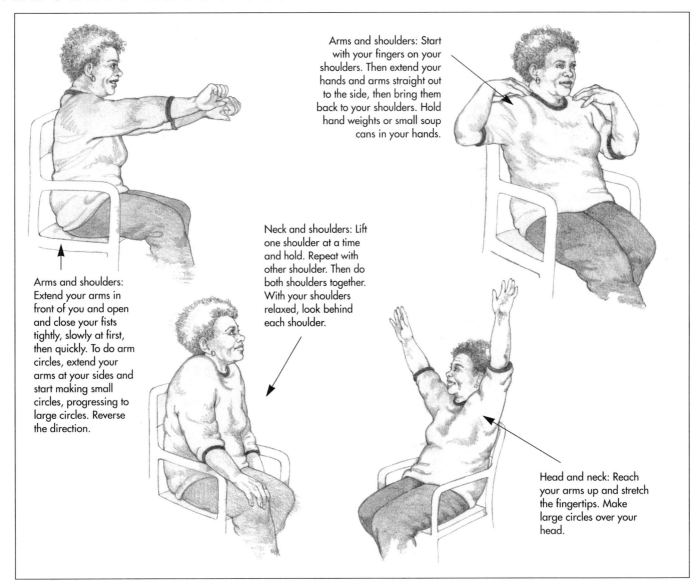

Arms and shoulders: Start with your fingers on your shoulders. Then extend your hands and arms straight out to the side, then bring them back to your shoulders. Hold hand weights or small soup cans in your hands.

Neck and shoulders: Lift one shoulder at a time and hold. Repeat with other shoulder. Then do both shoulders together. With your shoulders relaxed, look behind each shoulder.

Arms and shoulders: Extend your arms in front of you and open and close your fists tightly, slowly at first, then quickly. To do arm circles, extend your arms at your sides and start making small circles, progressing to large circles. Reverse the direction.

Head and neck: Reach your arms up and stretch the fingertips. Make large circles over your head.

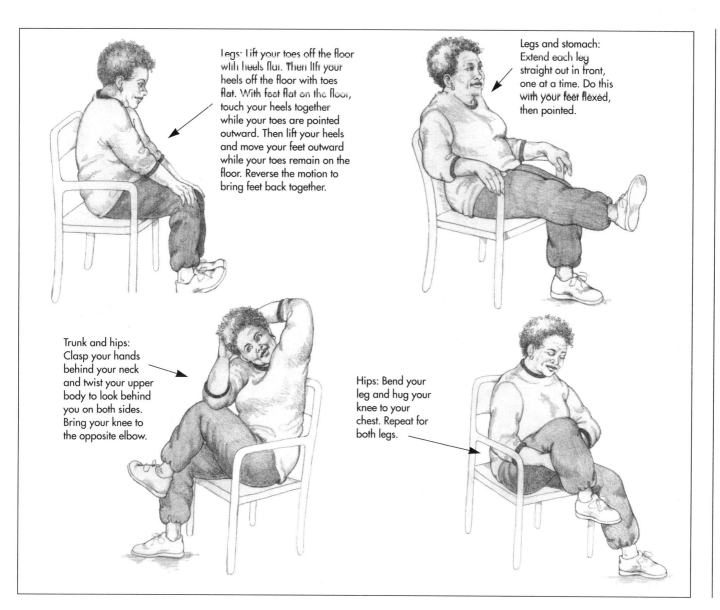

Legs: Lift your toes off the floor with heels flat. Then lift your heels off the floor with toes flat. With feet flat on the floor, touch your heels together while your toes are pointed outward. Then lift your heels and move your feet outward while your toes remain on the floor. Reverse the motion to bring feet back together.

Legs and stomach: Extend each leg straight out in front, one at a time. Do this with your feet flexed, then pointed.

Trunk and hips: Clasp your hands behind your neck and twist your upper body to look behind you on both sides. Bring your knee to the opposite elbow.

Hips: Bend your leg and hug your knee to your chest. Repeat for both legs.

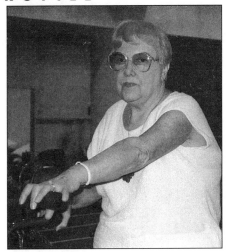

"I HAVE TO EXERCISE TO LIVE." Barbara Garman doesn't mince words. "I don't like exercise. I wouldn't do it for years." Now after 29 years of diabetes, Barbara, 68, says, "I still don't like exercise, but it's the key. You've got to do it."

Since Barbara has several serious diabetes-related complications, it may seem as though exercise would be out of the question. She suffers from both angina and neuropathy in her lower legs. Walking—the easiest, most inexpensive, and most accessible exercise—is not an option for Garman. Her neuropathy is so severe that she is virtually numb from her toes to her knees. She's been diagnosed with a broken toe and Charcot's foot and has had foot ulcers.

When Barbara's physician suggested she attend the Duke University Center for Living, she was more than willing. She

was ready to try anything to achieve a better physical quality of life. She and her husband, who does not have diabetes, spent three weeks at Duke, staying at a nearby hotel and attending the Center for Living programs during the day.

The Garmans have high praise for the Duke program, which includes a complete physical assessment, individualized treatment programs, and daily lectures. Her stay began with a physical examination. After the physical, the health-care team studied the results, examined her treatment program, and determined whether any changes were necessary. Then Barbara met with an exercise physiologist to plan an exercise program. Given the level of her diabetes-related complications, Barbara's physician would only approve a water exercise program and arm bicycling.

At Duke, Barbara and her husband joined the water walking class. In a large pool, the participants walk around the pool in one direction. Then they reverse directions, walking against the current they've created. Barbara learned how to check her pulse to make sure her heart rate was reaching her training range of 114 to 120 beats per minute. Although neuropathy has led to a lack of feeling in her hands, Barbara can feel the strong pulse in her neck. When water walking, Barbara walks for one hour and then cools down by doing stretching exercises in the water. Because the water supports 70 percent of body weight, stretching in the pool is easier on her entire body.

Barbara also learned how to do armchair stretches and to use an arm-bicycle machine at Duke.

Back home, Barbara and her husband had no problem continuing their water walking at a nearby health club pool. Unlike at Duke, Barbara and her husband are the only water walkers in the pool at home. At the end of her workout, Barbara—the nonexerciser—says she feels "invigorated and exhilirated, and I lost ten pounds over a few months."

In fact, when she returned from the Duke program, she had not only lowered her insulin dosage 16 units, but friends commented on how much more smoothly and easily she moved. But perhaps her strongest testament to the benefits of exercise comes from something that occurred during a trip to Florida. Before the Duke program, going up six or seven steps would bring on Barbara's angina. After the Duke program and several weeks of regular exercise, Barbara and her husband were staying on the sixth floor of a hotel, using the elevator. When the elevator broke down on the third floor, they got out and walked up to the sixth floor. Barbara walked up the three flights with no pain. She was so thrilled she told her husband she was ready to go back down and try it again.

Barbara Garman is the first to admit that exercise will never be her great passion, but she adds, "I have to exercise to live and to control my blood glucose...I have seen the results. Exercise really does work." ■

your feet or if you've had a leg or foot amputation, this can affect your balance. It can also affect how you place your feet on the ground. If it's hard for you to sense where your feet are, it is possible you'll misjudge when to place your weight onto them. You may find it helpful to exercise in front of a mirror so that you can see the position of your feet without moving your head. Exercises such as jogging and aerobic dance may not be right for you, because each time your feet hit the ground, they must withstand the full impact of your body weight. If your feet aren't ready to hold your body weight, you could be in for an injury. However, walking on a treadmill with handrails or using a stationary bike with handlebars may be possible. Another alternative might be chair exercises, especially if you are recovering from an amputation or have trouble walking (see pages 112 and 113). You'll be surprised how much these exercises can help you improve in strength and flexibility. Move to music and have a great time!

Exercises for people with peripheral neuropathy include those activities that don't put extreme stress on the legs, feet, or nearby joints. Bicycling is a great exercise because the bicycle supports your body weight and your feet can be kept in place with stirrups on the pedals. Rowing machines can be a good choice because they support your body weight and don't put an impact on your body. You should choose low-intensity rowing workouts. In other words, adjust the machine so that the resistance is low and you can row easily and comfortably without placing too much pressure on your feet.

If pushing with your feet is uncomfortable or unsafe, try working out with an arm-cycle ergometer. This is good for people who have undergone amputation or have limited use of their legs. Basically, it is a device that works much like a stationary bicycle, except that you use your arms to pedal instead of your legs. There are both free-standing and tabletop models.

Water exercise, which includes swimming or aqua aerobics (see above), can be done by almost anyone. The buoyancy of the water supports your body weight and provides enough resistance to improve strength and endurance. If you have an open wound, avoid working out in a pool until the wound heals. Be sure to wear shoes such as Aquasocks while you're in the water or around the pool to protect your feet.

You might be able to participate in outdoor activities where most of your muscular effort comes from the upper body. These include canoeing, rowing, and kayaking.

Autonomic neuropathy damages the nerves that control many involuntary body processes such as digestion, blood pressure regulation, and hormone secretions. Therefore, your body's normal control of blood pressure, hormone secretion, digestion, and the heart can be impaired during exercise. During exertion, you may not get enough blood to the extremities and brain, which may cause you to faint. So aerobic exercise may not be recommended. If you have been diagnosed with autonomic neuropathy, you should not exercise until your doctor and an exercise physiologist, if possible, approve a safe program.

If autonomic neuropathy has affected how well your body copes with the stress of exercise, especially how well the body senses and responds to low blood glucose levels, self-monitoring of blood glucose levels during exercise is absolutely necessary.

Exercises for people with autonomic neuropathy,

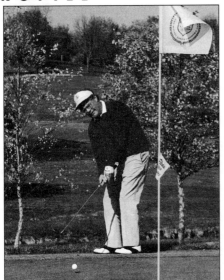

"NO ONE PREPARED ME FOR THIS PART."

Can people who have organ transplants actively exercise like everyone else? Yes! say 494 athletes from 34 countries who competed in the Eighth World Transplant Games in Budapest in 1993. Well, you may say to yourself, they're "athletes." What about me?

After three weeks of bedrest that can follow surgeries such as organ transplantation, everyone is down to zero on the fitness scale. In fact, says Burns Mossman, who received his kidney transplant in 1991, the simple act of taking a shower was so difficult that he had to sit and rest before he could undertake the "horrendous ordeal" of shaving. "No one prepared me for this part of the transplant." But he didn't let it keep him down for long.

Burns might fairly be described as a person who has type I diabetes and a type A personality. Burns has tackled diabetes head-on since the day he was diagnosed in February 1958 at the age of 14. He played football, basketball, and baseball in high school, earned his undergraduate and law degrees from the University of Iowa, and has made every effort to live an active and productive life.

He has dealt with several serious complications of diabetes, including severe retinopathy and circulation problems, but kidney failure demanded drastic measures. Burns received the kidney from his younger brother Mark. He was up walking within 16 hours of the surgery, but three weeks later he had to undergo a second, even longer surgery to move the kidney to the other side of his abdomen and to improve blood flow to it with a vein taken from his leg. Recovery from two surgeries and his kidneys not working for several weeks was slow, but by May 1992, Burns was back on the golf course.

Burns loves golf and being outdoors. "Missing three-foot putts is better than being in a hospital bed," he jokes. He rides a cart for most of the round, due to painful circulation problems in his legs and feet. For his aerobic workout, he rides a Schwinn Aerodyne stationary bike at home, especially during the winter months. Prednisone, an antirejection drug he has taken since the transplantation, has had an effect on his body, increasing his appetite and making his cheeks and body "rounder." Plus, the drug seems to encourage changes in muscle tissue. Burns considers these latest challenges minor in his determination to stay active and healthy every day of his life. As he says, "The transplant was the best option available, and the side effects are minor. I hope that this kidney lasts for the rest of my life. But if it were to fail, I would go through the whole transplant surgery again." ■

especially those with low blood pressure, include recumbent stationary cycling and aqua aerobics. Recumbent cycling involves pedaling a special stationary bicycle that allows you to recline at an angle rather than sitting up in a seat. Aqua aerobics uses the water pressure to help increase your blood pressure.

If you have autonomic neuropathy, you need to avoid activities that require rapid changes in body position such as aerobics or sports such as baseball, basketball, football, and tennis. You should also avoid exercising at a high intensity.

Retinopathy and vision loss.

Your blood glucose level can affect your vision. Some people report blurred vision when their blood glucose level is high. This is temporary and goes away when blood glucose levels go down. However, many years of high blood glucose levels can lead to diabetic retinopathy. Background retinopathy is especially common in people who have had diabetes longer than 10 years. In some cases, background retinopathy may need to be treated before you can exercise. In background retinopathy, fluid can leak from the retinal blood vessels. Because the retina is where the visual image forms, this damage can blur vision. Blood vessel damage is also related to high blood pressure.

If treatment is necessary, background retinopathy can usually be fully controlled with laser treatment by an ophthalmologist. For most patients, this means that after the treatment, they can resume or begin any exercises they would do otherwise. However, make sure your ophthalmologist gives you the go-ahead.

A more severe form of diabetic eye disease is called proliferative retinopathy. Exercising with untreated proliferative retinopathy is a serious threat to your vision. Proliferative retinopathy occurs when new blood vessels form on the surface of the retina. These actively growing vessels are fragile and easily broken, which can lead to bleeding and retinal detachment. Untreated proliferative retinopathy can lead to blindness. Proliferative retinopathy nearly always requires laser surgery.

Once blood vessel growth has been stopped with laser treatment and your retinopathy is considered stabilized, you will probably be able to return to or start your exercise program. Of course, you should make sure your ophthalmologist agrees that your eyes are ready. You may be advised to avoid stretching exercises that require you to lower your head below your waist. You may be told not to participate in contact sports, such as football or basketball. Make sure your ophthalmologist approves before you do scuba diving and high-altitude mountain climbing—the pressure changes involved can pose a risk to the blood vessels in your eyes.

If your vision is minimally impaired, don't despair. You still can benefit from aerobic exercise, and poor vision is not a reason to stop. You can ride a stationary bicycle or take a brisk walk on a treadmill. Row on a low-intensity rowing machine. Dance with a partner who can guide you. Be on the back end of a bicycle for two.

Water exercises are also great for people with low or partial vision. You can swim by guiding yourself with the touch of the pool's lane ropes. Or you can work out by doing aqua aerobics in the shallow water. If these choices don't appeal to you, ask your doctor or ophthalmologist for advice on how to perform your favorite workouts safely. There are blind snow skiers, water skiers, and bicyclists, so you are limited only if you believe you are.

Nephropathy and hypertension.

Nephropathy is a disease of the kidneys caused by damage to the small vessels or to the blood-cleaning units in the kidneys. Exercise itself does not affect kidney disease, but prolonged high blood pressure, such as hypertension, can bring on or worsen kidney disease. Because regular aerobic exercise can reduce high blood pressure, people with nephropathy are encouraged to exercise. If your doctor feels that your blood pressure is not a factor in your exercise program, let your personal tastes and overall fitness determine how you work out. Even if you are on dialysis, you can benefit from a slow, gradual, progressive exercise program.

If you have nephropathy and high blood pressure, you'll need to take a few precautions. You should have your doctor's approval on your exercise plans. Temporary high blood pressure can occur during high-intensity exercise, so avoid activities that are too strenuous for you. They will increase your blood pressure. If your workout feels too hard for you, it probably is. (This is true whether or not you have nephropathy.) You should not participate in competitive weight lifting. However, strength training using lower weights and many repetitions will help you develop strength and muscle mass. Make sure you receive training from an instructor on breathing and weight-lifting techniques so you can minimize the temporary increases in blood pressure that can occur during certain lifts. (See Resources for associations that certify strength trainers.) Holding your breath while you strain is not recommended. If you have questions about your limits, especially if you are concerned about blood pressure fluctuations, an exercise stress test will provide the answers.

If you choose long endurance exercises—such as aerobic exercise for longer than 45 minutes—that will cause you to dehydrate, drink plenty of water before, during, and after your workout. Don't wait until you feel thirsty.

Peripheral vascular disease.

This is a disease of the blood vessels in the arms, legs, and feet. Many people with peripheral vascular disease typically have an aching pain in their legs when they walk—a condition called *intermittent claudication*. This pain happens because the arteries in the legs occasionally close enough so that blood is unable to flow properly to the muscles that are being used. Typically, the pain occurs in the calves and feels like a cramping or aching sensation. Certain types of aerobic exercise such as swimming and bicycling help increase the circulation of blood, but discuss this type of exercise program carefully with your doctor before beginning. The medications you take may interfere with your ability to exercise. It is smart to avoid strenuous, high-intensity exercises such as sprinting or isometric weight lifting (when you keep your muscles contracted).

Interval walking is the best exercise choice for people with peripheral vascular disease and can be prescribed by your doctor as a nonsurgical therapy. To do interval walking, walk until pain in your legs or fatigue forces you to stop. Note how far you go; this is your maximum distance. The next day, walk three-quarters of the maximum distance you walked the day before. Rest a few minutes (until the pain subsides) and walk that same distance again. Walk three-quarters of your total distance three to four times each exercise session. Try to do this routine twice a day—such as once in the morning and once in the afternoon.

The second week, retest your maximum walking distance and repeat the interval training program. Every week, evaluate your maximum distance. Eventually, your walking periods will become longer and the rest periods will be shorter. A good goal is to increase the time, and therefore the distance, but not the intensity of your walk. By doing so, you'll improve the blood flow to the affected area. Soon you'll be able to walk pain-free for 30 to 45 minutes.

Atherosclerosis, heart disease, and hypertension.

Atherosclerosis (hardening of the arteries), hypertension, and heart disease are more common among people with diabetes and occur more often at a younger age. Because of this fact, if you are 35 years or older, you need a cardiac evaluation before you start an exercise program. If you have atherosclerosis, hypertension, or heart disease, you can benefit from an exercise program. But be sure to develop an individualized program with your health-care team.

Your doctor will probably advise you to take an exercise stress test (see Chapter 3). This test will help you and your doctor determine how healthy your heart is, what exercises you can safely do, and how much effort you can exert when you exercise.

Many people with heart disease or who are recovering from cardiovascular surgery are referred by their doctors to a cardiac rehabilitation program. This is a medically supervised program where your fitness level is tested and specific exercise (and sometimes lifestyle) recommendations are made. This is an excellent way to get back into an active lifestyle even with heart disease: The medical monitoring will build your confidence in your abilities and you will learn how to exercise safely on your own.

If you have hypertension or heart disease, avoid certain strenuous, high-resistance type exercises such as isometric weight lifting (keeping your muscles contracted) or exercises that involve pushing against an immovable object such as a wall. Moderate aerobic exercises (walking, low-impact aerobic dance, or leisurely bicycling) are better. You should limit exercise intensity to a heart rate that does not increase your blood pressure too high. You should not follow standard guidelines for target heart rate based on age, because you'll need to keep your blood pressure lower than most people while you exercise. The results of your exercise stress test will allow you and your health-care team to determine a safe heart rate range at which to exercise.

EXERCISE AFTER TRANSPLANTATION

Regular exercise should be a part of your recovery from kidney, pancreas, or kidney/pancreas transplantation. For most people, organ transplantation and weight gain go hand-in-hand, for two main reasons: usually your diet becomes relatively unrestricted, compared to your diet before transplantation, and your appetite increases because of prednisone, a drug that prevents organ rejection. Exercise will help you fight off this weight gain.

Prednisone also causes muscle wasting and weakness. Regular aerobic exercise and resistance (strength) training are the best ways to counteract this side effect of prednisone. It is especially important to progress gradually in aerobic and strength training, because prednisone may cause your muscles to adapt slower

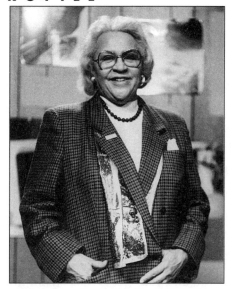

"YOU HAVE A GOOD HIGH." These days Barbara Lett-Simmons' schedule is so full, it's hard to find a few quiet minutes to chat. In addition to her volunteer duties with community organizations, she serves as president of her college alumni association and treasurer of the Washington, D.C. Mental Health Association. Recently appointed to the national council of the American Lung Association, she also serves as the local chapter president. Although she's been winding down her consulting business, she still provides training and development services to organizations in the Washington, D.C., area.

This level of commitment and activity is nothing new for Ms. Simmons. A former classroom teacher, education administrator, and 12-year member of the Washington, D.C. School Board, Ms. Simmons says, "I've always been a person of exceedingly high energy. I never walked. I was always at a half trot, taking stairs two at a time. When I taught, I used to race my children. I could always run faster."

Accustomed to feeling good and being on the go, she was at a loss to explain why several years ago, when she would sit down during the day, she'd doze off. She was seeing a doctor for peripheral vision loss in her left eye, when the answer emerged. Her vision problems stemmed from arteritis of the temporal artery of her left eye, but blood tests revealed another problem— diabetes. Suddenly, her daytime fatigue made sense.

Ms. Simmons was diagnosed with diabetes in 1991. Her approach to living with the disease is typically high energy and no nonsense. She learned to give herself shots from her physician's lab assistants and tests her blood glucose "every single day." Giving up sweets has been a struggle, she admits. But when she tests "there's a direct correlation. If I eat three cookies at night, I know that my glucose will be up there in the morning."

Ms. Simmons says she also sees

another direct correlation—between regular exercise and good blood glucose levels. Before she was diagnosed with diabetes, she'd started attending a water exercise class three times a week. She's stayed with the class and says it makes her feel "really good. I think it's like what I hear runners say about running—you have a good high. You feel good." She drives to the University of the District of Columbia pool for the Bodywise class, which is offered only to those 60 years and older.

For her eye condition, Ms. Simmons takes prednisone which caused a 50-pound weight gain. As her dosage has been reduced, she's been slowly taking off weight. To those who might be worried about their appearance in a bathing suit, Ms. Simmons is reassuringly down-to-earth. "Once you get to class, I don't care what your figure is, how wrinkled your skin is, how roly-poly your figure, there's always someone who looks worse than you!"

For those who flinch at the thought of entering a pool during the dead of winter, Ms. Simmons says, "the water is warm. You have showers. You have a locker room and ample room to dress and get comfortable." When she arrived for her first class, she found that she knew some of the people in the co-ed program. "It's good to have friends in class," says Simmons, "because you make each other go."

Although she's never had a problem with low blood glucose levels after exercise, she always carries crackers or lifesavers in her swim bag and keeps V-8 juice in her car.

According to Ms. Simmons, she's slowed down some. She no longer takes the stairs two at a time or races 6th graders across a school yard. Listening to the energy and enthusiasm in her voice as she talks about her volunteer work, her professional commitments, or her exercise program, there is no question. She's still a pacesetter. ■

"IT HELPS ME FEEL BETTER OVERALL."

A busy working mom with two children, Judy Mason tries to maintain a walking program to get regular exercise. Like many people, she finds it difficult to walk regularly in winter—it's dark after work and poor weather conditions can combine to make walking difficult and even dangerous. But in the spring, summer, and fall, Mason walks about two miles, three days or more a week. Usually she heads out to a high school track in her Washington, D.C., neighborhood. Sometimes her daughter rides along on her bike while Judy walks laps on the track.

As a benefits examiner with a pension agency, Judy's workdays often involve meetings and stress. She's says an evening walk is a good way to work off some of the day's tension, and she finds she enjoys the time to herself. "I'd rather not rely on someone else to exercise with. I'd rather go out on my own."

Judy likes walking because it's an inexpensive, convenient, and flexible way to get exercise. No special clothes or equipment are required, and you don't have to depend on anyone else to work out. Although Judy enjoys solo walks, she's also found attending a diabetes support group "very helpful."

Judy was diagnosed with type I diabetes at the age of 30. She's been attending support group meetings at Howard University Hospital in Washington, D.C., for two years. Judy says that her support group encourages regular exercise—sometimes the meetings even begin with a modest program of warm-up stretches. The meetings, which are normally attended by 25 to 30 people, offer "a lot of information that you don't normally hear about," says Judy.

Judy's blood glucose levels have always been pretty good, but she's quick to add that her walking program "helps me feel better over all. I do a lot of reflection and meditation [while walking]. I look forward to it." ■

than usual to exercise. An aerobic workout of 30 to 45 minutes at a moderate intensity is a good goal.

If your transplantation surgery is uncomplicated, you should start trying to walk after just a few days. If you have significant weakness in your leg muscles, start some low-intensity strengthening exercises as soon as you can. For instance, work out with therabands (large rubber bands with varying amounts of resistance) and progress to light weights to prevent muscle shrinkage due to disuse. If you have trouble walking, try pedaling a stationary bike. Cycling will help build your endurance without you having to support your body weight. Keep working on building up your time spent walking, however. Walking works the muscles that support your body.

EXERCISE AND PREGNANCY

Many women continue to exercise during pregnancy, and for good reason. Exercise during pregnancy helps you maintain your level of fitness, moderate weight gain, increase strength and stamina, and decrease back stress and anxiety. Being physically fit can make the burden of pregnancy easier to bear and will prepare you for the work involved with labor.

If you are a regular exerciser with type I or type II diabetes, you've come to depend on how exercise lowers your blood glucose level. Now is the most important time to keep your blood glucose level as normal as possible. If you've developed gestational diabetes during pregnancy, exercise can help you lower your blood glucose level and so is an effective part of the treatment plan.

Despite the benefits, however, exercise poses risks for women who are pregnant. Therefore, if you are pregnant, consult with your doctor before exercising. Following the American College of Obstetricians and Gynecologists (ACOG) recommendations, you should definitely not begin a new strenuous exercise program during pregnancy, particularly if you weren't a regular exerciser before pregnancy. However, your doctor together with your obstetrician might suggest that you begin a new low-intensity program. Regular exercisers can usually keep exercising during pregnancy, with their doctor's and obstetrician's okay.

Based on your medical history, your doctor and your obstetrician should help you develop a safe exercise routine. They will take into consideration your diabetes control, your age, complications, medications, and the length of time you've been pregnant.

ACOG recommends the following exercise guidelines for women who are pregnant.

- Regular exercise is better than occasional workouts.
- Warm up before and cool down after exercise to prevent injuries.
- Don't overstretch or perform bouncing, jerky movements or quick changes in direction. As ligaments and joints progressively relax to prepare for growth and delivery of the baby, you are more susceptible to joint and ligament injuries.
- Drink plenty of fluids before and after exercising. Pregnancy increases your risk of dehydration.
- Your heart rate should not go above 140 beats per minute during exercise (around 23 beats in a 10-second pulse).
- Don't allow the strenuous part of your exercise routine to last longer than 15 minutes. As stren-

uous exercise time goes up so does the risk for injuries. You can participate in lower intensity exercises, such as walking, for up to 45 minutes. Stop exercising if pain or unusual symptoms appear.

Avoid the following:

- Exercise that involves lying on your back after your fourth month of pregnancy
- Exercise that involves straining or holding your breath
- Exercise that involves jerky movements
- Activity that causes rises in your core body temperature above 100 degrees, such as exercising in extreme heat or taking saunas or whirlpool baths longer than 10 minutes—a rise in internal body temperature can harm the baby.

It is crucial to your and your baby's good health that you manage your blood glucose levels. You will be asked to keep blood glucose levels as normal as possible, which can mean you may have more episodes of hypoglycemia. You need to frequently test your blood glucose level, particularly before and after you exercise. You and your health-care team will need to work together to make specific plans for your blood glucose control during exercise. Keep an exercise log.

You will need to eat additional calories to cover the exercise you plan to do. This will also help you avoid exercise-related hypoglycemia. Because tight control of blood glucose level is crucial, your doctor or dietitian should help you decide what foods and how much of them you should eat to cover your exercise plans.

Some good exercises during pregnancy include recumbent cycling, swimming (lap swimming and aqua aerobics), and walking. Working out with an arm-cycle

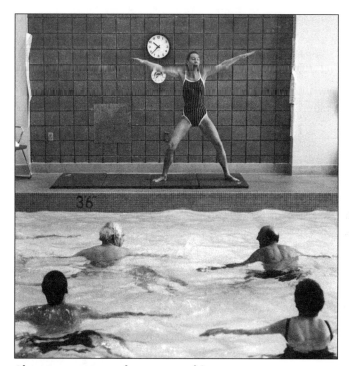

Almost anyone can do aqua aerobics.
Photograph by Les Todd, courtesy of Duke University Photo Department.

ergometer is a good way to get an aerobic workout with upper body exercise. Ask your obstetrician to show you how to palpate your uterus to detect contractions that can signal that you're overdoing it. This is especially important in the third trimester. Activities to avoid include scuba diving, water skiing, platform diving, high-altitude mountain climbing or skiing, gymnastics, volleyball, and horseback riding. Your health-care team should help you determine the best exercises for you. You will be able to continue your exercise program after your baby is born and while you are breastfeeding. ❧

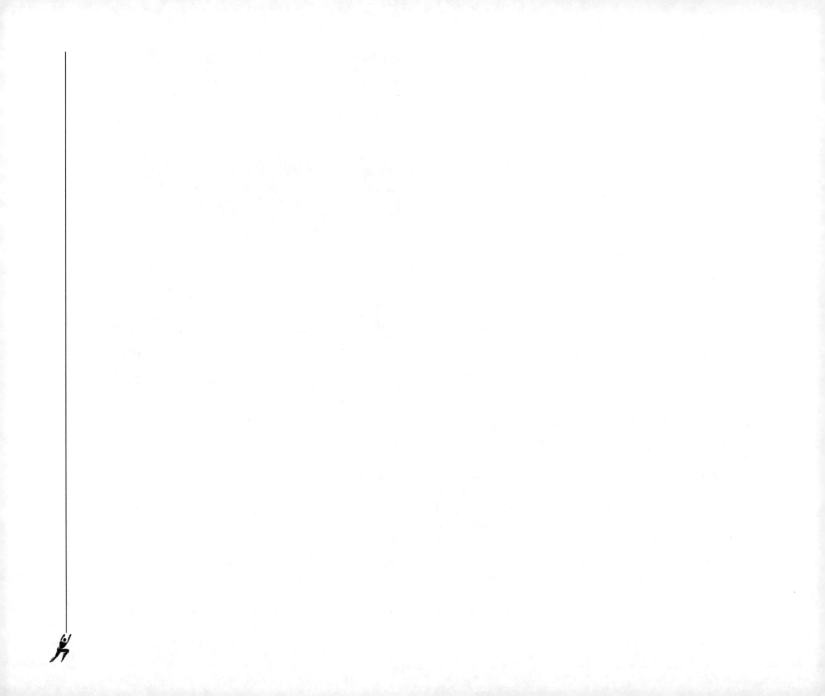

I would rather be ashes than dust! I would rather my sparks should burn out in a blaze than be stifled by dry rot. I would rather be a superb meteor, every atom of me in magnificent glow than asleep on a permanent planet. The proper function of man is to live, not to exist. I shall not waste my days trying to prolong them. I shall use my time.
—Jack London

Competing With Diabetes

AFTER A YEAR OF REGULAR JOGGING, YOU'RE WONDERING ABOUT TACKLING A 10K RACE. Or perhaps you love softball and have been thinking about joining the team at work. Or maybe you're a ten-year-old trying out for the swim team. If you've been getting fit for a while, chances are at some point you're going to want to compete. Whether you're competing against your own personal best effort or working with teammates to capture a title, competition offers some great rewards. It's a terrific way to stay motivated, challenge yourself, and grow. It's also a good way to meet others with similar interests.

Does diabetes stand in the way of competition? Athletes from former hockey star Curt Fraser to National Football League stars Jonathan Hayes and Wade Wilson to golf champion Sherri Turner have shown that, when it comes to athletic competition, having diabetes doesn't put you out of the game. Athletes with diabetes of all ages and skill levels enjoy competing in their chosen sports. For some athletes, diabetes was a way of life long before entering competitive sports. Others were already professional athletes when diagnosed.

DO YOU HAVE WHAT IT TAKES?

Having diabetes teaches us skills. Luckily, the skills needed to maintain good blood glucose control are identical to the skills needed for athletic success. You're probably already equipped with

- Desire to do the job right. The successful athlete is committed to doing the job right by continually learning and modifying training. Optimum blood glucose control takes a similar straightforward commitment to life-long learning about diabetes and the willingness to make lifestyle adjustments as necessary.
- Knowledge of how the game is played. To be the best athlete possible means knowing the game inside and out. Similarly, taking charge of your diabetes care means having a thorough understanding of how the disease works and how exercise and diet affect your diabetes.

- Discipline to play by the rules. Just as players must abide by the rules of the game, the athlete with diabetes needs the discipline to methodically monitor blood glucose levels, avoid unhealthy food choices and activities, and routinely opt for healthy alternatives.
- Skill. For all athletes, experiencing your "skill" at an activity is immediate, gratifying feedback. It's also a great motivator. Once you've achieved an athletic goal, chances are you'll push yourself ahead. Maintaining optimum blood glucose levels requires not only technical skill but the willingness to challenge yourself to do better.

TEAM SPORTS

Whether you are an eight-year-old soccer standout who's just been diagnosed, a college athlete who's been insulin-dependent for a year, or a 50-something tennis player who's had type II diabetes for 10 years, team sports can be an important part of your life. If you enjoy working with teammates toward a common goal, having diabetes doesn't relegate you to the sidelines. Here's what you need to have to participate:

- Reasonably good control: exercise puts you at risk for hypoglycemia and hyperglycemia, but you can minimize the risks.
- Freedom from diabetes complications that may hinder your participation: your preexercise exam results have already told you whether you need to cross some sports off your list because of high blood pressure, proliferative retinopathy, or heart disease.
- Good communication with your health-care team, coach, and teammates.

Regardless of your age or athletic ability, you, the athlete with diabetes, are the only one with the knowledge and ability to control your day-to-day changes in blood glucose levels. If you are a young player, you may need to do this with the help of your parents and coach.

What your coach needs to know.

The relationship between a team player and coach depends on many factors. Obviously elementary and middle school-age players will have a different relationship with their coach than a high school or college athlete. For the professional athlete, the relationship is different as well.

Your coach will need to know:

■ what diabetes is
■ your ability to play despite having diabetes
■ how you handle your diabetes: how you plan ahead to avoid getting hypoglycemia and when you are likely to test your blood glucose.

For the younger player, the coach may need to have a role in testing blood glucose and helping treat a hypoglycemic reaction. Depending on your circumstances, you may want to have your doctor, parents, and coach talk about specific issues.

What your parents need to know.

Children with diabetes can and should enjoy a range of sports activities. Your child will probably let you know the extent of his or her interest and enthusiasm for an activity. Your child has many role models of successful athletes with diabetes such as 1950s tennis pro Bill Talbert and 1990s NFL quarterback Wade Wilson.

This is not to minimize the frustrations and anxiety that are part of the athletic equation for any parent. Strenuous exercise can make blood glucose levels more difficult to control. When children start traveling to out-of-town meets, parental anxiety can soar. But, among other things, competitive athletics can give your child a chance to make new friends, develop physical confidence, and improve self-esteem.

To help your child have the best possible sports experience:

■ build strong lines of communication with your child's health-care team.
■ talk with other parents of children with diabetes.
■ look for new sources of information and support for athletes with diabetes, such as the International Diabetic Athlete's Association (see Resources).
■ explain diabetes to your child's coach, but let your child handle telling teammates.

HOW DO YOU SEE YOUR DIABETES?

One thing that seems to unite successful athletes with diabetes is attitude. They view diabetes not as a barrier to competition but as a factor to be dealt with. Careful planning, good support from your health-care team, good communication with coaches and teammates, and the ability to make changes in your diabetes management routine when necessary will allow you to compete on any level from recreational to professional.

The late George Sheehan, MD, runner, philosopher, and author, wrote that each athlete is an experiment of one. This holds especially true for the athlete with diabetes. You know your body's response to activity better than anyone else. Intense exercise, especially the kind of effort required in competition, can make controlling blood glucose levels more challenging.

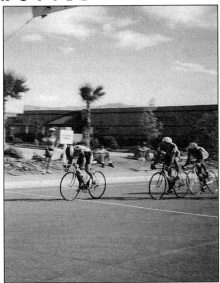

"I'M SUPER, SUPER COMPETITIVE."

Asked to describe himself as an athlete, competitive cyclist Jeff Monken says "I hate to lose. When I'm riding my bike, I don't like people passing me. It really gets my blood flowing. I'm super, super competitive. I like being the best."

Monken, a 29-year-old district sales manager from Oceanside, California, began bike racing about two and a half years ago. A soccer player in college, Monken was diagnosed with diabetes the day before his final exams senior year. "I just thought I've been through too much [getting through college] to let diabetes keep me from living my life. It was a major shock, but the more I thought about it the more I thought, it's not that bad. It's manageable. If I'd been diagnosed 25 years ago, I could have died."

After college, Monken played racquetball and ran, but knee problems led him to try cycling. Bike racing fit Monken's competitive spirit to a tee. It's the rush of adrenalin that he loves. "Once you get in that pack of 100 guys, it really gets exciting," he says.

Monken competes in criterium races. For a criterium, a one- or two-mile course is laid out, usually in a business park. The riders repeat this loop 15 to 20 times, racing a total distance of between 20 and 30 miles. Criteriums are strategic races, involving close cooperation among cycling team members. Monken rides for the Celo Pacific Racing Team.

"You really get involved with your teammates," says Monken. "Because they can help you in a race, you really learn how to work together. You learn about position. You learn where to be at what time."

"Everyone I ride with knows I have diabetes. I've never had a problem on my bike, but I want them to know." Coincidentally, two of Jeff's teammates also have type I diabetes.

Although diabetes has never caused a problem on his bike, it did wreak havoc with Jeff's racing efforts. "Last year I didn't place or win any races. I raced the whole season—26 races—but never had the control I needed." Frustration set in. "From the amount of exercise I was doing I wasn't able to keep my blood glucose levels up consistently. I was having problems with low blood glucose and my performance was hampered. To compensate I actually got my blood glucose too high some times. I couldn't stay level."

Then a profile of exercise physiologist Claudia Graham, PhD, in Diabetes Forecast led him to a diabetes management program in Century City, California. A health-care team helped him resolve his exercise-induced blood-glucose problems.

"First they did a VO_2 max test. Then they went through my diet and training program. I went for an initial visit and then I kept a diary of everything for one month—everything I ate and drank, and my exercise. And, I checked my blood glucose three times a day for a month."

When he returned to the center, they put him on a training program for one month. Monken says the center changed the way he was taking insulin, the amount, and the way he ate. They also worked with him on different sports drinks to use during longer rides—such as 100-mile training rides. He now uses a sports drink that gives a quick replacement for carbohydrates lost once he's depleted the glycogen stored in his muscles.

Jeff credits the program, which reworked his exercise prescription to fit his specific needs as a competitive cyclist, with salvaging his racing. "This program made the difference. I was stagnant in racing and losing some interest because I wasn't progressing."

The racing season runs from March through October. During the season, Jeff rides about 250 miles per week. In the off-season, his mileage drops in half. This year, with the changes in his diabetes management, Jeff has seen a dramatic improvement in his racing. In the 1992 season, he won six races, and his ranking was upgraded to catgory 3, which allows him to compete in the Nationals.

Jeff credits his diabetes with helping him to be a winner. "I'm healthier. I eat better. Plus diabetes has gotten me involved in cycling, which I enjoy. It's really caused a lot of good things in my life." ■

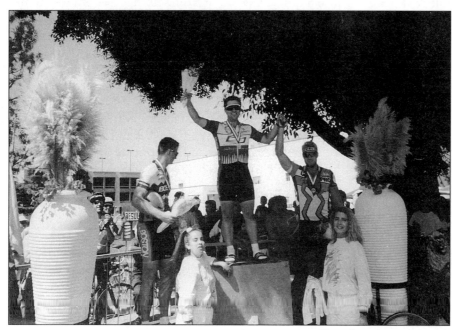

Jeff on the winner's stand.

For each person with diabetes, the effects of exercise and exercise intensity are individual. An individualized treatment plan is critical to your athletic success. Developing the optimum balance of food, exercise, and medication will take some trial and error.

No one system works for all athletes. Workouts are sport specific—you don't train for competitive swimming in the same way you train for a soccer match or for running a 10K race. Your chosen sport will dictate many of the factors that influence your diabetes regimen. Is your sport seasonal? Is it aerobic (swimming or running) or anaerobic (weight lifting, sprinting, or baseball)? Do you follow a set training schedule that peaks for competition? Is your main competitive effort a single event or a series? Does your sport impose weight requirements like gymnastics or wrestling? Are you coming back from an injury? You will need to have access to the advice of your health-care team, especially your doctor and dietitian, to keep your diabetes management program in balance with all the factors affecting your training.

As an experiment of one, you will need to work out the diabetes management routine that best meets your body's exercise expenditures. Flexibility and optimal blood glucose control are essential to successful athletic competition for those requiring insulin. Although this book provides a basic framework of information, examples of what has worked for other athletes, and suggestions of important considerations, you'll need to take matters into your own hands. As you ask your body for optimum athletic effort, you will be creating your personal diabetes management plan.

THE KEYS TO ATHLETIC SUCCESS

While no one system works for every athlete, most successful competitive athletes with diabetes have several things in common:

- They test their blood glucose levels frequently.
- They keep a training log.
- They have an individualized treatment plan they hammered out through trial and error.
- They have developed an ability to be flexible in their approach to diabetes management and athletic training.

To these athletes, frequent self-testing is a boon rather than a burden. It's an expensive routine, but it is also a quick way to buy yourself the freedom to pursue your goals. When NFL star Jonathan Hayes describes a typical game day, he reports testing before and after the game. You, too, need to test your blood glucose level before and after activity. You may also want to monitor during the activity, particularly if it's a long event, for example, if you're involved in morning-long playoff competition. But don't stop there. You also need to know what the numbers mean and what to do about them.

Scuba instructor and diver Steve Prosterman says he likes to know which way his blood glucose level is headed before a dive. To find out, he tests about one hour before, 30 minutes before, and then immediately before a dive. By comparing the numbers he knows whether his blood glucose level is headed up or down and what precautions to take. If he's heading down, even if the latest reading is in the safe zone, he'll have a snack before diving.

Do you know your warning signs for hypoglycemia? Don't ignore them if you want to keep going. Some people who've had diabetes for many years no longer feel the classic warning signs of hypoglycemia. If this is true for you, try to tune into other signs of possible hypoglycemia, and test. You will need to monitor your blood glucose levels for several hours after exercising, when hypoglycemia is most likely to appear.

A training log can be the best resource you have. It lets you see your progress and helps you analyze setbacks. A training log can be an important tool in understanding how exercise and competition are affecting your control.

Your log can be formal or informal. Bookstores sell specially designed runner's logs, or you can use a notebook or desk calendar. You can adapt one of the exercise logs found in Chapter 4.

A log is the best resource you can offer your health-care team in your efforts to fine tune your diabetes management program. When competitive cyclist Jeff Monken's racing went through a flat spell, he decided to go for a complete reevaluation of his diabetes management program. The medical team he worked with asked him to keep a precise account of his workouts, his insulin dosages, and everything he ate and drank for one month. This information, along with some additional exercise testing, helped his health-care team rework his diet and insulin dosages. The result was better control, and he started winning races!

When you set a new athletic goal, such as running a marathon, you'll need to revamp your training program. To do this, you must have the flexibility to make changes in your diabetes treatment routine and the resources to individualize your program. This means that you need to know how diabetes affects your body and how you can,

with food, exercise, and medication, affect your blood glucose level. The information you record in your training log will be vital when you and your health-care team try to troubleshoot and reevaluate aspects of your diabetes management program such as insulin dosages or dietary changes.

FUELING UP

In their drive to excel, elite athletes leave nothing to chance. In recent years, there has been increasing interest in the interaction between nutrition and athletic performance. Seeking every possible advantage, athletes look to good nutrition to give them the competitive edge. After all, food is the fuel for competition. The good news

---

TABLE 1

GENERAL GUIDELINES FOR FOOD INTAKE FOR EXERCISE

- If blood glucose is under 100 mg/dl before exercise, eat a preexercise snack.
- If blood glucose is 100 to 150 mg/dl, go ahead and exercise, but retest during your workout if you plan to exercise longer than 30 minutes and a eat snack afterward, if necessary.
- If blood glucose is higher than 250 mg/dl:
    - If you have type I diabetes, test urine for ketones; if ketones are moderate or high, usually this means you need more insulin; do not exercise until ketone levels are negative or trace.
    - If you have type II diabetes, go ahead and exercise, unless your doctor has told you to test for ketones and follow guidelines for type I diabetes.

TABLE 2

FOOD GAME PLAN

■ Pregame meal: Eat this one to three hours before starting time.

■ Aim for: A meal high in carbohydrates, some protein, and a minimum of fat.

■ Food choices: Lean meat, fish, or poultry; potatoes without gravy; pasta with tomato sauce; vegetables; bread (no butter); salad with fat-free dressing; fruit and skim milk.

■ Drink: Remember to drink water or another fluid before the event. Have three or four cups of fluid with your meal and drink again before the event.

■ Pregame snack: You may need to add a snack of fresh fruit or fruit juice immediately before the game.

■ During the game: For long and intense activity, you may need to supplement with carbohydrate every 30 to 60 minutes. Sports drinks or diluted fruit juices may work for you.

■ Afterward: You may need a postgame snack of carbohydrate to ward off exercise-induced hypoglycemia later.

energy, glycogen stored in your muscles breaks down into glucose. This glucose, in turn, provides more fuel for exercise. The trick is, the storage of carbohydrate as glycogen requires insulin. So, good diabetes control is important to allow your body to both use and store carbohydrates. Eating before, during, or after strenuous exercise may be important for everyone who exercises, but it's essential if you have diabetes (Table 1). Review your meal plan with your dietitian to find out whether you are eating the carbohydrates you need. You may want to try out the game-day food plan found in Table 2.

Plan ahead to avoid hypoglycemia. If you use insulin, you have the added worry of hypoglycemia during competition. Eating a small amount of carbohydrate before or after exercise can help prevent blood glucose level from going too low. Although avoiding hypoglycemia may be your biggest immediate concern, keep in mind your long-term goal of keeping blood glucose levels close to normal to avoid diabetes complications. The Diabetes Control and Complications Trial results showed that tight blood glucose control gives you your greatest chance for avoiding diabetes complications. The best way to decide whether you need extra food to cover your energy expenditures is by monitoring your blood glucose level and discussing the results with your doctor and dietitian. Do some experimenting and find out what snacks or sports drinks work best for you before, during, and after exercise to keep your blood glucose levels within a safe range.

You may not need extra food before exercise. This decision depends on your blood glucose levels before

for people with diabetes is that the optimum meal plan for you is the one nutritionists recommend for most athletes—a diet high in carbohydrates and low in fat with adequate amounts of protein.

For an athlete with diabetes, a nutritious eating plan has two aspects: it helps fuel your exercising muscles, and it helps you control your blood glucose levels.

Strive for good control. Regularly eating a diet high in carbohydrates helps promote glycogen storage. Carbohydrates are stored as glycogen in the muscles and liver. As you exercise and your body demands more and after exercise, how close the exercise is to a scheduled meal and snack, and how often you exercise. The more regularly you exercise, the more your body adapts. If you're working out on a regular basis, snacks should be a part of your meal plan. You will want to work closely with your dietitian to fine tune your meal plan to meet your exercise expenditures and help you toward your athletic goals.

Don't forget your water bottle. It's easy to become dehydrated while exercising. Sometimes it's obvious that you need to drink, as you sweat through a summer workout. Other times, training for a swim meet or sailboarding in a cool breeze, it may slip your mind. Dehydration causes you to lose coordination. It can also lead to heat cramps, heat exhaustion, and even heat stroke. Distance runners frequently hear the maxim don't wait until you're thirsty to drink. Athletes with diabetes may be so focused on the need to replenish their carbohydrate stores, that they forget the first nutrient needed by all exercisers: water (Table 3).

CARBOHYDRATE REPLACEMENT

Replacing carbohydrates used during exercise is important. Stress hormones stimulate the release of glucose from stored glycogen for use during the beginning of exercise. Studies report that when people without diabetes exercise with moderate intensity for more than one and a half to two hours, blood glucose levels begin to drop. In people with diabetes, this blood glucose drop can happen sooner and can progress to hypoglycemia if carbohydrates aren't consumed. Studies report that taking some form of carbohydrate during this period extends your ability to keep on going.

Although everyone needs carbohydrates during exercise, for athletes with diabetes, consuming 10 to 15

T A B L E 3

HOW TO STAY WET WHILE COMPETING

It's important to replace fluids lost during exercise.

- Note weight changes during workouts in your training log. Drink two cups of water for every pound lost during exercise.
- Hydrate before your competition. Two hours before an event, drink 2 to 3 cups of cold water, and 10 to 15 minutes before beginning, 1 or 2 cups of additional water. Cold water is absorbed faster by the body than warm water.
- Try to drink 1/2 to 1 cup of water at 15- to 20-minute intervals during the event.
- Once you pass the one-hour mark, drink a sports drink or some diluted juice to replace carbohydrates as well as fluids lost.
- After your workout, remember to drink again. You should regain weight lost through sweat, and your urine should again be pale in color.
- Hydrate during training. During an event, water is usually plentiful. If you train informally or by yourself, it's easy to forget to drink, especially in cool weather. Plan ahead. Stash water bottles along your running route if public fountains aren't available.

Adapted from Franz MJ: Fuel for exercise. *Diabetes Forecast* 46: 30–33, 1992

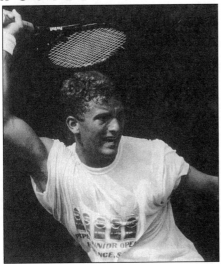

"I TEST SO MUCH BECAUSE MY SCHEDULE IS SO ERRATIC."

For Chris Robinson, 1984 was a year to remember. Although he was 11, it was the year he began competing in national tennis tournaments. It was also the year he was diagnosed with type I diabetes.

Since then, Chris has continued to hone his tennis skills. In 1990, he was rated among the top 50 players in his age group nationwide and was number one in the Mid-Atlantic region.

As a 19-year-old sophomore, Chris completed his second year at Clemson University on a tennis scholarship. The Clemson program, one of the most rigorous in the country, relies on physical conditioning. But following a disciplined routine is something very familiar to Chris Robinson.

Just how tough is the Clemson program? Consider this: freshman and upperclassman who cannot run a mile in 5:15 when training season starts go through an initial two weeks of "morning madness." This means running for an hour and a half every morning, topped off by trotting up some stadium steps. Once they're up to speed, the team does weight training two or three times a week, and, yes, plays tennis, too.

Chris stays on top of his game by following a disciplined schedule and diet. He takes four or five shots a day and usually tests his blood glucose level six or seven times daily. "The reason I test so much is my schedule is so erratic with so much exercise at weird times. I have to test a lot—before I run or before a match."

In his sophomore year, tennis team members all lived in one dorm, and Chris ate in the college dining hall. He says he could find the variety of foods he needed. His diet, then and now, emphasizes complex carbohydrates and avoids sugars and fats. Breakfast and lunch are primarily made up of bread and cereals, along with some fruit, and dinner is a well-balanced meal that includes all the food groups. On match day, Chris doesn't vary his diet, but supplements with a fluid-replacement drink designed for athletes or orange juice courtside.

After all these years on the court, what keeps Chris motivated? "Probably the thing that fires me up the most is being able to compete well. To do a lot of things to let other people who would be intimidated by diabetes know that it's nothing to be scared of. I thank God for the ability he has given me to play tennis." ■

"I WAS COMPLETELY FOCUSED ON THE DAILY CHALLENGES."

For recreational cyclist Meg Richter, biking is something more than a good way to get an aerobic workout. "I've always enjoyed cycling. I find it relaxing and challenging. I don't think of it as exercise. There's definitely an exercise element, but there's more to it than that," she says. The "more" she's talking about is the feeling of relaxation and freedom she gets rolling through the suburban Philadelphia countryside. During the good-weather months, she averages about 100 miles a week.

Meg, 35, has had type I diabetes for 13 years. Her love of cycling predates the diagnosis. "Now I'm sort of graduating from doing a lot of cycling on my own to going out with a group," she says. "I just decided it was time to learn more technique and to improve my riding speed." Meg is a member of the Bicycle Club of Philadelphia. One way Meg's working to improve her cycling is by riding with a group that's "just a little above my level."

In terms of cycling, Meg finds having a goal helps. "It helps me push myself to go toward it," she says. One goal Meg achieved was cycling from Philadelphia to Atlantic City (62 miles). Several years ago, friends were planning the ride. Meg says, "At first I thought, I can't do it, because of my diabetes. But the next spring I thought, who says I can't do that?" Meg recalls. She completed the ride not once, but several times since then.

In the summer of 1991, Meg set herself another challenge. She signed up for an Outward Bound course in Maine. The program involved hiking, backpacking, canoeing, and much more. All Outward Bound programs offer participants physical challenges in an environment of group support. "I'm not a person who is comfortable with taking physical risks, and for me this was a risk," says Meg. First, she pushed herself to get into shape for the course. She opted for a course offered to adults with diabetes. The coed group ranged in age from early 20s to 40s. Meg says the fact that everyone had diabetes worked to create a uniquely supportive environment. "I wasn't so intimidated. I could stop when I wanted to test or eat a cracker. The program provided a kind of relaxation that I haven't experienced since I got diabetes. With diabetes you have to constantly monitor yourself. You can't skip it if you're tired or don't feel like it—it's not like brushing your teeth or washing your face. The constant listening to your body is a strain. We had to do that at Outward Bound, but I really forgot about the diabetes, because I was completely focused on the daily challenges at hand. It was very relaxing.

None of us was the odd person out." Meg says, whatever your goals, Outward Bound helps you challenge yourself and take risks, while making you feel safe.

Riding with her new club, Meg admits to some self-consciousness. But, she says, things are working out well. "A lot of these rides have their own break points, and I can stop and test. I'll just do it, and people will ask, 'What are you doing?' I'll say that it's a machine that tests my blood glucose. I don't bother to hide it, but I don't go into a lengthy explanation. I figure if they want to know more, they'll ask."

During long rides, she checks her blood glucose every hour or hour and a half. She packs carefully beforehand. Supplies she brings on long rides include glucose tablets or glucose gel, food bars, and testing supplies. If her blood glucose is under 200 before the start of a ride, she usually eats something. "I'm probably more cautious than I need to be," says Meg, "but that makes me feel safe. By doing that, I can concentrate on the ride and not be distracted by worries about my blood glucose." ■

grams of carbohydrate after about every 40 to 60 minutes of exercise (and if you continue to exercise, doing this each additional hour) is very important. For very intense exercise or competitive activities, you may need 10 to 15 grams of carbohydrate every 30 minutes. For long periods of exercise, the amount of food needed may be substantial. It may not be desirable or practical to increase your food intake to accommodate your energy expenditures. Instead, you may need to reduce your insulin dosage.

Fruit juices diluted with water and most sports drinks (see below) are good sources of both fluid and carbohydrates during and after exercise. They provide fuel, help control body temperature, and can also help keep blood glucose levels in an appropriate range. The reason they work well is that they are diluted carbohydrates, which are rapidly absorbed. If you use a sports drink to replace lost carbohydrates, look for one with less than 10% carbohydrate. If the carbohydrate is too concentrated, such as regular fruit juice or regular soda, which contain 12% or more carbohydrate, the body cannot absorb it as quickly. Concentrated carbohydrates can cause stomach cramping, nausea, diarrhea, bloating, and discomfort. If you choose fruit juice or regular soda, you'll need to dilute it with an equal amount of water (1/2 cup juice with 1/2 cup water) so it can be absorbed more quickly.

Not only can appropriate carbohydrate replacement help prevent hypoglycemia during exercise, it can also help avoid hypoglycemia after exercise. Foods containing carbohydrates and that are low in fat are your best bet for snacking. Good choices include low-fat crackers, muffins, yogurt, soups, peanut butter and crackers, fig bars, oatmeal-raisin cookies, dried fruit,

bread sticks, and granola bars. Fruits such as apples, peaches, pears, and plums have natural sugars, vitamins, and minerals and are 85% water.

Have you been tempted to buy special diets, vitamin and mineral formulas, and "power boosters" to increase your athletic performance? Unless your diet lacks a particular vitamin or mineral, you will not benefit from these quick fixes. Your body is built primarily by exercise, not by diet supplements. If you're not where you want to be with your current training routine and you have extra resources to spend on boosting your performance, consider consulting an exercise physiologist and/or a dietitian.

These guidelines provide you with the big picture: the importance of eating nutritious foods, staying hydrated, and replacing carbohydrates during exercise. But as an athlete—an experiment of one—you will need to test and modify your program. You may find one sports drink works better for you than others. Perhaps a certain pregame meal suits you physiologically and psychologically. A ritual of a specific snack may be just what you need. You are the best interpreter of your body's signals. To compete at your optimum level, you'll need to become an expert in reading and responding to them. You may even enjoy the challenge as much as the competition.

HIGH-RISK SPORTS—A PERSONAL CHOICE

The question is no longer whether people with diabetes can or should participate in high-risk sports. In fact, people with diabetes can and do. It's more appropriate to ask what is the safest way to enjoy these activities? And under what circumstances is a high-risk sport just a plain bad risk?

Sports that fall into the high-risk category include

scuba diving, sea kayaking, mountain climbing, rock climbing, backcountry hiking, sky diving, prize fighting (boxing), hang gliding, and auto racing. The decision to pursue a high-risk sport is personal. Participating means that you are accepting a level of risk at the outset. If you enjoy a so-called high-risk sport, you obviously do not want your diabetes to make the venture riskier.

Steve Prosterman, Diving Supervisor/Captain for the University of the Virgin Islands, has had insulin-dependent diabetes since 1966. He's been a scuba diving instructor since 1982, and he is a paramedic in the St. Thomas Decompression Chamber, which is used to treat diving accidents. Steve also enjoys sailboarding, surfing, sea kayaking, and ocean swimming. In 1990, Steve began running a camp for people ages 17 to 23 with diabetes. During the camp program, he teaches scuba diving, sailboarding, sea kayaking, and sailing.

For Steve, high-risk sports are a way of life. But, by careful planning and following explicit safety rules, he might argue that he's vastly reduced the risk factors involved. Steve is direct about the fact that water sports present additional problems for people with diabetes. During many of these activities, he points out, participants are isolated on or under the water.

Safety is his first priority. Hypoglycemia is a real concern for those interested in high-risk water sports, he says. If you have poorly controlled diabetes or are subject to unpredictable bouts of hypoglycemia, high-risk activities are not recommended. If you are in good control and take some extra precautions, Steve maintains that diabetes is not a barrier to safe diving. He also reports that you can get scuba certification, if you find an instructor willing to teach you and a doctor willing to give you medical clearance. Although the absolute

limit to scuba sports diving is 130 feet deep, someone with diabetes should go no deeper than 60 feet of water. A condition called nitrogen narcosis, which creates a state of confusion and altered consciousness, can occur at depths deeper than 60 feet and hide or add to an episode of hypoglycemia.

Here are Steve's guidelines for participating in high-risk water sports. They can be applied, with sensible changes, to any high-risk sport where you are isolated. You need to have:

■ well-controlled diabetes. In general, well-controlled diabetes would mean having a glycated hemoglobin near normal. This range is usually 4 to 7 percent, sometimes 8 percent depending on the lab. A glycated hemoglobin reading in this range indicates that your day-to-day control has averaged out near normal.

■ freedom from complications that would indicate the activity should be avoided.

■ the ability to recognize hypoglycemia in its early stages and treat it by yourself.

You also need to be willing to do a little more.

■ Steve not only tests immediately before a dive, he also tests about one hour and a half hour earlier. This allows him to know the direction in which his blood glucose level is headed. His blood glucose may be 140 right before the dive, which is fine, but if it had been slightly elevated earlier, these tests would indicate that his blood glucose level was falling. He would eat an extra snack and then test again to make sure that blood glucose level isn't still falling. Steve also tests after a dive to see what effect the dive had on the blood glucose level.

■ You and those around you need to be able recognize when you are in the early stages of hypoglycemia and know how to treat it.

- You should always carry some form of quick-acting carbohydrate. Steve and his students always carry at least four tubes of glucose gel into the water, two in their bathing suits and two in their scuba gear. He cautions that water, especially, salt water, destroys packaging. You need to plan ahead. Steve has found InstaGlucose packaging holds up well against salt water. Others report success with Monogel. Or you can carry your supplies in a water-proof bag or bottle with a waterproof seal.

- Plan ahead for taking carbohydrates while on the water, if necessary, to treat or avert a hypoglycemic episode. Scuba diving presents some extra challenges. Diving buddies practice the hand signals indicating low blood glucose (or another reason to surface) before they begin the dive. If carbohydrates are needed, Steve teaches his students to come to the surface with their buddy or group, inflate the buoyancy compensator, eat their carbohydrate snacks, terminate the dive for the time being, and if possible, do a blood test.

- For events of long duration, test your blood glucose during the activity. Dives are relatively short—30 minutes to an hour. However, sea kayaking and sailboarding may mean being out for hours. It is possible to come in to test or to test on the water if you have a waterproof bag for your meter. Water destroys meters, however, so you need a dry spot to test.

- If in doubt, err on the side of going high when you are on the water.

The Hurricane Island Outward Bound school offers another approach for those wanting to try some high-risk activities within a framework of group support. Since 1987, Raymonde Herksowitz Dumont, MD, senior clinic physician at the Joslin Diabetes Center, has been conducting Outward Bound courses for people with diabetes. The first course—a sailing course—was aimed at teenagers with diabetes. Based on the success of the initial course, Outward Bound and Dr. Dumont planned a course for adults. Since then, Dr. Dumont and the Hurricane Island Outward Bound staff have had at least one adolescent and one adult course per year.

Self-discovery is an inherent part of the Outward Bound experience. It pushes people in their level of self-care because the circumstances under which they are asked to provide care are tough. Accomplishing tasks like rock climbing or a ropes course or navigating unknown territory plus taking care of your diabetes can lead you to see that in daily life, you can find time for good diabetes management.

Dr. Dumont, who is an assistant clinical professor of pediatrics at Harvard University Medical School, has been both the health-care professional and a co-instructor in each of these programs. Participant safety is a foremost concern, but Outward Bound courses also encourage self-reliance as well as group support. Although participants do not have to be in excellent physical condition, the course does require a bare minimum of fitness. There is no age limit set for the adult courses. The youngest participant was 15, the oldest 52.

Steve Prosterman's work in the Virgin Islands and Hurricane Island Outward Bound School's courses for people with diabetes are just two examples of approaches to high-risk sports that have succeeded for people with diabetes. ❧

AEROBIC EXERCISE:
Activities of moderate intensity that use large muscle groups and require increased oxygen intake for sustained periods.

ANAEROBIC EXERCISE:
Activities of high intensity that can be performed for only short periods.

CARDIOVASCULAR ENDURANCE:
The ability of the heart, lungs, and circulatory system to supply oxygen and nutrients to working muscles for long periods.

CIRCUIT WEIGHT TRAINING:
A series of weight-training exercises performed with minimal rest in between (15 to 30 seconds) before moving from one exercise to the next.

FITNESS: Combination of aerobic health, muscular strength and endurance, flexibility, and healthy body composition.

FLEXIBILITY: The range of motion possible in a joint or series of joints.

FREE WEIGHTS: Weights that are free from cables or other devices that restrict their movement, such as dumbbells and barbells.

HEART RATE: The number of heart beats in a minute, measured by counting the pulse.

MET: A unit of resting energy expenditure. A person exercising at 4 METs is burning four times the number of calories as at rest.

MUSCULAR ENDURANCE:
The ability of a muscle or group of muscles to contract for some extended period of time at a nonmaximal force.

MUSCULAR STRENGTH:
The maximum force a muscle or group of muscles can produce.

REPETITION (REP):
The number of times you lift a weight at one sitting.

SET: A group of repetitions make up a set. If you perform 8 repetitions during one lift that would be one set of 8 reps.

VALSALVA MANEUVER:
Straining while holding your breath.

VO₂ MAX: Maximum oxygen uptake possible by the body, usually measured in millimeters of oxygen per kilogram body weight per minute. This defines a person's capacity for aerobic exercise.

WEIGHT LOAD: How many pounds you lift. If you lift 20 pounds, your weight load is 20 pounds.

WEIGHT MACHINES:
These are machines that are guided by levers, cables, or chains. Nautilus, Cybex, and LifeCircuit are well-known names in weight machines.

ASSOCIATIONS OF SPECIAL INTEREST

Your best resource for information is likely to be your local American Diabetes Association Affiliate, listed in the white pages of your telephone book.

AMERICAN DIABETES ASSOCIATION

1660 Duke Street
Alexandria, VA 22314
(800) 232-3472
The nation's leading organization helping people with diabetes. As a member, you'll join more than 270,000 people with diabetes in supporting research to prevent and cure diabetes and programs to help people with diabetes live better. Through your American Diabetes Association Affiliate, you'll have access to support groups, classes, and other services.

The resources listed below may offer important additional services and/or information.

INTERNATIONAL DIABETIC ATHLETES ASSOCIATION

6829 North 12th Street, Suite 205
Phoenix, AZ 85014
(602) 230-8155
Members are people with diabetes interested in being active at all levels and health-care professionals. Gives basic guidelines on nutrition and sports, practical advice for specific conditions, quarterly newsletter, and national and international annual meetings. Promotes networking, support, and sharing of experiences.

THE AMERICAN DIETETIC ASSOCIATION

216 West Jackson Boulevard, Suite 800
Chicago, IL 60606
(312) 899-0040
(800) 877-1600
Members are professional dietitians. Provides information, guidance, and referrals to local professional dietitians.

PRESCRIPTION FOOTWEAR ASSOCIATION

9861 Broken Land Parkway, Suite 255
Columbia, MD 21046-1151
(800) 673-8447
Can refer you to a local certified pedorthist (someone trained in fitting prescription footwear).

OUTWARD BOUND

384 Field Point Road
Greenwich, CT 06830
(203) 661-0797
(800) 243-8520
Operates 5 wilderness schools and 6 urban centers in the United States to help young people and adults discover and extend their own resources and abilities by confronting them with a series of increasingly difficult challenges. Courses for people with diabetes. Programs operate in 22 states and other areas, including Kenya, Nepal, and Russia.

CAMP DAVI

(809) 774-9907
(809) 776-2885
With the University of the Virgin Islands, the Diabetes Association of the Virgin Islands (DAVI) sponsors a yearly 1-week camp for people with diabetes ages 17 and older who want to try scuba diving, snorkeling, sea kayaking, sailing, and sailboarding.

ORGANIZATIONS THAT CERTIFY EXERCISE PROFESSIONALS

To find an exercise physiologist, contact your health-care delivery system, local hospitals, county medical centers, or local universities, or ask your physician or diabetes educator for a referral.

AMERICAN COUNCIL ON EXERCISE
5820 Oberlin Drive, Suite 102
San Diego, CA 92121-3787
(800) 529-8227
Certifies and conducts training and continuing education for aerobics instructors and personal trainers. Gives local referrals.

AEROBICS AND FITNESS ASSOCIATION OF AMERICA
15250 Ventura Boulevard, Suite 310
Sherman Oaks, CA 91403
(818) 905-0040
Certifies and conducts training and continuing education for aerobics instructors. Confirms whether your instructor is certified, but does not give referrals.

AMERICAN COLLEGE OF SPORTS MEDICINE
PO Box 1440
Indianapolis, IN 46206-1440
(317) 637-9200
Certifies fitness instructors, exercise specialists, and exercise test technologists; offers continuing education. Publishes books and pamphlets for professionals and patients. Confirms whether your instructor is certified, but does not give referrals.

AQUATIC EXERCISE ASSOCIATION
PO Box 497
Port Washington, WI 53074
(414) 284-3416
Holds educational events and workshops, certifies aquatic exercise instructors, gives referrals to local certified instructors; serves as resource for services and products.

NATIONAL STRENGTH AND CONDITIONING ASSOCIATION
PO Box 81410
Lincoln, NE 68501
(402) 472-3000
Operates professional certification program. Individuals may write for addresses of local certified professionals, include draft of letter, pay fee.

PROFESSIONAL ASSOCIATION OF DIVING INSTRUCTORS
1251 East Dyer Road, No. 100
Santa Ana, CA 92705
(714) 540-7234
(800) 729-7234
Educates and certifies underwater scuba instructors. Sanctions instructor training nationwide and in 87 countries. Provides course criteria, training aids, and requirements for all aspects of diving instruction.

UNITED STATES WATER FITNESS ASSOCIATION
PO Box 3279
Boynton Beach, FL 33424
(407) 732-9908
Promotes activities such as water aerobics, water walking, water running, and deep water exercise. Certifies water fitness instructors and program coordinators and gives local referrals.

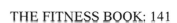

ORGANIZATIONS THAT PROMOTE SPECIFIC SPORTS

AMATEUR ATHLETIC UNION OF THE UNITED STATES (AAU)
3400 West 86th Street
PO Box 68207
Indianapolis, IN 46268
(317) 872-2900
Sponsors AAU/USA Junior Olympic Games; Chrysler Fund-AAU Physical Fitness Program, AAU Youth Sports Program, and the Presidental Sports Award.

AMERICAN VOLKSSPORT ASSOCIATION
Phoenix Square, Suite 203
1001 Pat Booker Road
Universal City, TX 78148
(210) 659-2112
Provides information about walking and other noncompetitive organized sports activities and recreation programs for all ages.

AMERICAN YOGA ASSOCIATION
3130 Mayfield Road, W-103
Cleveland Heights, OH 44118
(216) 371-0078
(800) 226-5859
Teaches classical yoga with emphasis on breathing, exercise, and relaxation/meditation. Has specially designed programs for the elderly ("Easy Does It Fitness"), which include workshops for health professionals and other fitness trainers throughout the country.

BLIND OUTDOOR LEISURE DEVELOPMENT, INC.
533 East Main Street
Aspen, CO 81611
(303) 923- 3811
Assists blind people in appreciating outdoor recreation. Aids local clubs in developing programs in skiing, skating, hiking, fishing, horseback riding, swimming, and biking.

FELDENKRAIS GUILD
524 Ellsworth Street
PO Box 489
Albany, OR 97321-0143
(503) 926-0981
Teaches physical movements to coordinate brain and body for improved performance, and ease in movement. Ideal for people with discomfort with physical activities, pain, or chronic conditions.

NASTAR/NATIONAL STANDARD RACE WORLD WIDE SKI CORPORATION
402-D, AABC
Aspen, CO 81611
(303) 925-7864
Administers the National Standard Race (NASTAR) program for Ski magazine. Gives everyday skiers a chance to race gates for practice, for fun, and for a score. More than 4 million skiers of all ages and abilities have competed against their previous score, their neighbor's score, and the handicap set by the fastest member of the U.S. Ski Team.

NATIONAL HANDICAPPED SPORTS ASSOCIATION
451 Hungerford Drive, Suite 100
Rockville, MD 20850
(800) 966-4647
(301) 217-0960
Promotes sports and recreation opportunities for individuals with physical disabilities. Offers year-round programs in most sports including learn-to-ski, learn-to-sail, and learn-to-race clinics, special programs for children, women, and veterans with disabilities.

NATIONAL ORGANIZATION OF MALL WALKERS

PO Box 191
Hermann, MO 65041
(314) 486-3945
Individuals engaged in fitness programs involving walking through shopping malls. Sponsors walking events and fitness promotional programs. Bestows distance awards.

NATIONAL SENIOR SPORTS ASSOCIATION

10560 Main Street
Fairfax, VA 22030
(703) 385-7540
Men and women 50 years of age and older interested in sports and recreational activities. Helps improve and maintain physical and emotional well-being through organized sports and recreation. Conducts golf and bowling tournaments.

NATIONAL WHEELCHAIR ATHLETIC ASSOCIATION

3595 East Fountain Boulevard, Suite L-1
Colorado Springs, CO 80910
(719) 574-1150
Members compete in various amateur sports events in wheelchairs. Annual National Wheelchair games at local, regional, and national meets include track and field, swimming, archery, shooting, table tennis, and weightlifting.

PRESIDENT'S COUNCIL ON PHYSICAL FITNESS AND SPORTS

701 Pennsylvania Avenue NW, Suite 250
Washington, DC 20004
(202) 272-3421
Encourages regular participation in sports and physical fitness activities for people of all ages. Information, brochures, and awards for individuals (and teams) of all ages.

SOCIETY OF SAUNTERERS, INTERNATIONAL

2461 Whitehouse Trail
Gaylord, MI 49735
(517) 732-2547
Seeks to inform dedicated walkers, inspire new walkers, and motivate nonwalkers to walk. Believes that walking is the greatest and most lasting activity for physical and mental well-being. Provides information on the creative, ecological, medical, philosophical, and spiritual benefits of walking; current events in walking; and walking themes.

UNITED STATES BLIND ATHLETES ASSOCIATION

33 N. Institute Street
Bryan Hall, Suite 015
Colorado Springs, CO 80903
(719) 630-0422
Promotes sports for the legally blind and visually impaired athletes. Organizes regional, national, and international competitions. Sports include skiing, goalball, gymnastics, judo, powerlifting, speed skating, swimming, tandem cycling, track and field, and wrestling.

UNITED STATES CYCLING FEDERATION

1750 East Boulder
Colorado Springs, CO 80909
(719) 578-4581
Governing body of amateur cycling in the United States. Supervises and controls all amateur bicycle competitions; promotes safety education. Bestows awards, keeps records, and runs training camps and clinics.

UNITED STATES ROWING ASSOCIATION

201 S. Capitol Avenue, Suite 400
Indianapolis, IN 46225
(317) 237-5656
For individuals who are competing rowers, former rowers, and rowing enthusiasts. Promotes, governs, and fosters amateur rowing in the United States.

UNITED STATES MASTERS SWIMMING

2 Peters Avenue
Rutland, MA 01543
(508) 886-6631
Adults aged 19 years and older interested in participating in swimming for fun, fitness, and competition. Sponsors competitions, research, and educational programs.

U.S. NATIONAL SENIOR SPORTS ORGANIZATION

14323 S. Outer Forty Road, Suite N300
Chesterfield, MO 63017
(314) 878-4900
Promotes fitness, healthy lifestyles, and participation in athletic competition for people over 55 years old. Holds biennial multisport competitions (next games 1995); bestows awards.

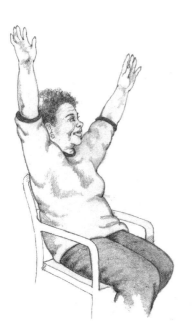

OTHER HELPFUL ORGANIZATIONS

AMERICAN AMPUTEE FOUNDATION

PO Box 250218
Hillcrest Station
Little Rock, AR 72225
(501) 666-2523
Provides information to amputees and other disabled people, including those with spinal cord injuries, about services, equipment, and support groups.

NATIONAL INSTITUTE ON AGING INORMATION CENTER/EXERCISE

PO Box 8057
Gaithersburg, MD 20898-8057
Write for Elder Fit and Mature Stuff, and other fitness information for older adults.

TRANSPLANT ATHLETES GAMES SPONSORED BY THE KIDNEY FOUNDATION

(800) 622-9010
For information about the national and international transplant athlete games and athletic rehabilitation after transplant surgery.

BOOKS OF INTEREST FROM THE AMERICAN DIABETES ASSOCIATION:

For information on how to order these publications, call the ADA at (800) 232-3472, ext. 363.

TYPE II DIABETES: YOUR HEALTHY LIVING GUIDE

The first all-in-one sourcebook for managing type II diabetes. New ideas, practical suggestions, gives you all the ways to live healthy with diabetes.

EAT FOR LIFE

The nine-point dietary plan to reduce your risk of diet-related diseases, presented using sensible guidelines without measuring or calculating. "How-to" section offers tips on shopping, cooking, and eating out.

NECESSARY TOUGHNESS

by Jonathan Hayes with Robert Briggs. Autobiography of Jonathan Hayes who developed diabetes in college and went on to successfully play professional football.

GRILLED CHEESE AT FOUR O'CLOCK IN THE MORNING

Ages 8–12. Charming novel reassures and encourages children with diabetes to cope like Scott, the main character in the book, who discovers some important lessons about himself—and life.

DIABETES & PREGNANCY: WHAT TO EXPECT

Comprehensive guide for women with type I diabetes. The specifics are covered in detail: the stages of an unborn baby's development, tests to expect, labor and delivery, and birth control.

GESTATIONAL DIABETES: WHAT TO EXPECT

The guide that helps you learn what gestational diabetes is and how to care for yourself during your pregnancy.

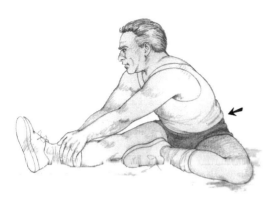

FROM OTHER PUBLISHERS:

AQUACISES: RESTORING AND MAINTAINING MOBILITY WITH WATER EXERCISES

Miriam Study Giles. Miles & Sanderson, Bedford, MA 01730. To order, write Miles & Sanderson, Publishers, 41 North Road, Suite 201, Bedford, MA 01730-1021. Instructions for anyone, but especially seniors or those with handicaps, on how to keep active with pool workouts. (800) 441-6224 orders only.(617) 275-1410.

AWESOME TEEN

Chris Silkwood and Nancy Levicki. NJL Interests, Houston, TX. To order, write to Awesome Teen, 7714 Woodway, Dept. A, Houston, TX 77063. Smart choices for teens who are interested in body image, health, diet, and fitness.

LIVING WITH EXERCISE: IMPROVING YOUR HEALTH THROUGH MODERATE PHYSICAL ACTIVITY

Steven N. Blair. Am Health Pub. Co. Dallas, TX. To order write the Learn Education Center, 1555 West Mockingbird Lane, Suite 203, Dallas, TX 75235. For anyone interested in exercise for health. Stresses moderate activity, explains "moderate," and gives quizzes and checklists.

RUNNING & BEING: THE TOTAL EXPERIENCE

by George Sheehan, MD. Simon and Schuster, New York, NY. The famous cardiologist, columnist, and runner shares his philosophy of exercise, of running, and of being. Thoughts to round out your workout.

STRETCHING

Bob Anderson. Shelter Publications, Bolinas, CA. To order, write the author at PO Box 279, Bolinas, CA 94924. The complete guide to improving your flexibility and workouts with stretching.

THE ATHLETE'S GUIDE TO SPORTS PSYCHOLOGY

Dorothy Harris, Human Kinetics Publishers, PO Box 5076, Champaign, IL 61825-5076, (800) 747-4457. Mental conditioning is as important as physical conditioning—use mental imagery to practice your form or a particular skill. Learn to relax, turn off the mind chatter, and focus on your athletic performance. ■

INDEX

A Aerobic capacity; See VO_2 max
Aerobic dance, 70–71
Aerobic exercises, 33–35, 40t, 66, 96–97, 118; See also Machines, exercise
aqua aerobics, 70, 110, 115
bicycling; See Bicycling
capacity for, testing, 22–23
cross-country skiing, 72
dancing; See Dancing
fitness and, 65–72
high-impact, 70
jogging, 67
low-impact, 70
running, 67
swimming, 67–70, 110, 115, 118
walking, 66–67
for weight loss, 96–97
American Diabetes Association, 32
Angina, 19
Animal insulin, 59t
Aqua aerobics, 40t, 70, 110, 115
Aquasocks, 70, 110, 115
Arm-cycle ergometers, 115, 123
Arm exercises, 73–74, 112
Arteries, hardening of, 25, 119
Atherosclerosis, 25, 119
Athletes, professional; See Competitive sports
Athletic clubs/gyms, 89–90
Autonomic neuropathy, 23, 115–117
Auto racing, 137

B Baseball, 96
Basketball, 108–108, 117
Beginners, weight reduction and, 93–97
Bench aerobics, 70–71
Bicycling, 40t, 71, 84–85, 110, 115, 118; See also Stationary bicycles
Blood glucose levels, 2–3, 5
controlling, 47–61; See also Insulin
and carbohydrate replacement, 58t
and competitive sports; See Competitive sports
and diet-managed diabetes, 60–61
hyperglycemia and; See Hyperglycemia
hypoglycemia and; See Hypoglycemia
ketosis and, 49–52
pregnancy and, 123
self-monitoring, 18, 52–56
tailored plans, 57–58
"tight" control, 5, 57, 93, 123,132
warning signs and, 59–60
fasting, 21t
monitoring, 3, 43
postmeal, 21t
response to exercise, 57
Blood lipid levels, 5, 6
Blood pressure, 6, 22, 36
high; See Hypertension
low, 19
Blood tests, common values for, 21t
Blood vessel disease, 3, 5, 18–19
Body fat composition, 15–16, 25–30
Body weight; See also Weight control/reduction
diabetes and, 92–93
Boxing, 50, 137

C Calories, 123; See also Aerobic exercises; METs
burning, 92
and diet changes, 99–103
Canoeing, 115
Capillary beds, 5
Carbohydrates, 58t, 62, 133–136, 138
Cardiac rehabilitation programs, 119
Cardiovascular disease; See Heart disease
Chair exercises, 110–111, 112–113
Cheerleading, 34
Cholesterol, 5–6, 21t
Circulation, in feet, 62–64
Clothing, 64
Coaches, diabetes awareness and, 127–128
"Comfort zone", exercise program design and, 35–41
Competitive sports, 125–138
basketball, 108–109, 117
and blood glucose control skills required, 126
carbohydrate replacement and, 133–136
cycling, 128
fluids and, 132
high-risk, 136–138
nutrition and, 131–133
running, 28–29, 88, 94–95
success in, 127–131
swimming, 56
team sports, 126–127
Complications of diabetes, 5–6, 18–21, 36, 111–119, 126, 132
Contact sports, 117
Cool-down routines, 61
Cross-country skiing, 40t, 72
machines for, 87
Cross-training, 15, 103
Curl-ups, 75

D Dancing, 40t, 70–71, 115
Dehydration, 62, 133
Diabetes
background on, 2
and body weight, 92–93
competition and; See Competitive sports

complications of; See Complications of diabetes
inherited, 6
insulin-dependent (type I); See Insulin-dependent diabetes
non-insulin-dependent (type II); See Non-insulin-dependent diabetes
"tight control" versus standard control, 5
Diet
changing, 99–103
and diabetes management, 60–61
diet history, 22
and non-insulin-dependent diabetes, 46, 60–61
Dietary supplements, 136
Dieting, problems with, 97–98
Disuse syndrome, 106
Duration, of exercise, 41

E Energy cost of exercise, 40t
Equipment, for exercise programs, 9; See also Machines, exercise
Exercise
American Diabetes Association guidelines for, 32
benefits of, 2–5
diabetes complications and; See Complications of diabetes
duration of, 41
energy cost of, 40t
exertion levels and, 35–41
and fluid intake, 61–62, 133, 136
frequency of, 41–42
hunger and, 97
and injuries; See Injuries
intensity of, 35–41
medically supervised, 89, 110, 119
mental preparation for, 7–16
METs and, 40–41

persistence in, 14–16
physical preparation for, 17–30
planning, 31–46
and pregnancy, 122–123
program assessment, 8–14
record keeping and, 42–46
safety during, 47–64, 106
self-motivation and, 8, 14–16, 103
types of, 33–35, 66
Exercise logs, 43–46, 131
Exercise testing, 22–30
body fat composition measurements, 25–30
flexibility tests, 23–25
stress tests, 22–23
Exertion, levels of, 35–41
Expenses, of personal exercise programs, 14
Extremities; See Peripheral vascular disease
Eyes
examinations of, 22
small blood vessel disease and, 3, 5; See also Retinopathy

F Feet, problems with, 62–64
Flexibility, 23–25, 35, 76–83
Fluids, 61–62, 133, 136
Food, competition and, 131–133
Football, 96, 117
Frequency, of exercise, 41–42
Fruit juices, 62, 136

G Glycated hemoglobin, 19, 21t
Goals, for exercise programs, 15–16, 20t, 33
Golf, 96
Gyms/athletic clubs, 89–90

H Hang gliding, 137
HDL cholesterol, 5–6, 21t

Heart disease, 3, 5, 18–19, 22, 36, 119
Heart rate, 119
resting, 66
target, 36–39
estimating, 38
Hemoglobin, glycated, 19, 21t
High-density lipoprotein (HDL) cholesterol, 5–6, 21t
High-risk sports, 136–138
Home equipment; See Machines, exercise
Home workouts, 90
Human insulin, 59t
Hunger, exercise and, 97
Hyperglycemia, 2, 3, 27, 49–52, 126
Hypertension, 5, 11, 19, 83, 117–119
Hypoglycemia, 48–49, 126, 130–132, 136, 137
intensive insulin therapy and, 93
pregnancy and, 123
recognizing, 59–60

I Inactivity, 96–97
Infections, foot, 62
Injuries, 9, 11, 19, 68, 93, 110, 122–123
aerobic dance and, 70
avoiding, 35, 59, 61
bicycling and, 71
cross-country skiing and, 72
duration of exercise and, 41
flexibility and, 76–77
running/jogging and, 67
strength training and, 76, 111
swimming and, 70
walking and, 66
Insulin, 18, 33, 92–93; See also Blood glucose levels, controlling
action of, 58–59
efficient use of, 3
as "storage hormone," 2

Insulin-dependent diabetes, 2–3, 5, 18, 33
  ADA exercise guidelines and, 32
  and exercise logs, 44
  hyperglycemia and, 49–52
  hypoglycemia and, 48–49
Insulin reactions, preventing, 53t
Insulin resistance, 2, 6, 25, 92–93
Insulin sensitivity, 6, 41
Insulin therapy, 43
  intensive, 93
Intermittent claudication, 19, 118
Interval walking, 118–119
Isometric weight lifting, 118, 119

J Jogging, 40t, 67, 96, 115

K Kayaking, 115, 137
Ketoacidosis, 52
Ketosis, 3, 18, 44–46, 131t
  and blood glucose control, 49–52
  self-testing for urine ketones, 55
Kidneys, 3, 5
  transplantation, 119–122

L Large blood vessel disease, 3, 5
LDL cholesterol, 5–6, 21t
Leg exercises, 73, 113
Lifestyles, exercise programs and, 11
Low-density lipoprotein (LDL)
  cholesterol, 5–6, 21t
Lung capacity; See VO$_2$ max

M Machines, exercise, 83–88
  choosing home equipment, 83–84
  cross-country skiing machines, 87
  rowing machines, 86–87
  stair climbers, 85–86
  stationary bicycles, 84–85
  treadmills, 85
  VCRs and, 87–88

Medication, 118
  and ability to exercise, 18
  heart rate and, 107
Metabolism, 2; See also Diet
METs, 40–41
Motivation, 8, 16, 103
Mountain climbing, 117
Muscles
  building; See Strength training
  loss of, dieting and, 98
  stretching; See Flexibility

N National Strength and Conditioning
  Association, 11
Native Americans, 100–101
Nephropathy and hypertension, 118
Nerve damage, 19, 21, 62, 111–117
Neuropathy, 62, 111–117
Non-insulin-dependent diabetes, 2–3, 5, 6, 8, 18, 33
  ADA exercise guidelines and, 32
  and body weight, 92–93
  diet-managed, 60–61
  exercise logs and, 45–46
  heredity and, 6
  hyperglycemia and, 49–52
  hypoglycemia and, 48–49
  preventing, 6
Nutrition, competition and, 131–133

O Obesity, 2, 6, 15–16, 96
Oral hypoglycemic medications, 2, 43, 45
Outward Bound, 138
Overload principle, 32
Oxygen consumption; See VO$_2$ max

P Pancreas, 2, 3
  transplantation, 119–122
Parents, team sports and, 127
Peripheral neuropathy, 111–115

Peripheral vascular disease, 118–119
Personal health history, 18–19
Physical exams, 11, 18–22
Physical limitations, 11
Physical preparation, for exercise, 17–30
  exercise testing and, 22–30
Physiologists, exercise, 30
Prednisone, 119–120
Preexercise physicals, 18–22
Pregnancy, 122–123
Prevention, of non-insulin-dependent diabetes, 6
Proliferative retinopathy, 117
Protein (muscle), loss of, dieting and, 98
Push-ups, 75

R Rating of perceived exertion (RPE), 39
Record keeping, 43–46
Resistance training; see Strength training
Retinopathy, 22, 83, 117
Risk factors; See Complications of diabetes
Rock climbing, 137, 138
Rowing, 115
Rowing machines, 40t, 86–87, 115
RPE (rating of perceived exertion), 39
Running, 40t, 41, 67, 96

S Safety
  blood glucose levels and; See Blood glucose levels, controlling
  during exercise; See Exercise, safety during
Sailboarding, 137
Sailing, 137, 138
Schedules, for exercise, 14–15
Scuba diving, 117, 130, 137–138

Seasons, exercise and, 11
Self-monitoring, 130
  blood glucose levels, 18, 52–56
  ketone levels, 55
Self-motivation, 8, 14–16, 103
Senior citizens, 105–111
  bicycling and, 110
  chair exercises for, 110–111,
    112–113
  and walking, 107
  water exercises and, 110, 115
Shoes, 63–64, 71
Sit-and-reach test, 25
Sit-ups, 75
Skinfold tests, 26–27
Skydiving, 137
Small blood vessel disease, 3, 5
Smoking, 19
Socks, 64
  Aquasocks, 70, 110, 115
Specialists, 22–30
Special needs, 105–123
Specificity principle, 32
Sports drinks, 62, 136
Stair climbing, 35, 41, 85–86
Stationary bicycles, 40t, 84–85,
  100–101, 122
Step aerobics, 70–71
"Storage" hormones; see Insulin
Strength training, 11, 35, 118, 122;
  See also Machines, exercise
  and fitness, 72–76
  isometric, 118, 119
  for senior citizens, 111
Stress tests, 22–23
Stretching, 61, 76–82
Strokes, 5
Supplements, dietary, 136
Support networks, 14–15
Swimming, 40t, 67–70, 110, 115, 118,
  123

T T'ai Chi (Taijiquan), 83
Tapes (video), for fitness training,
  87–88
Target heart rate, See Heart rate,
  target
Team sports, 126–127; See also
  individual sports
"Tight control" of diabetes, 5, 57,
  93, 123, 132
Training, 9–11, 15
Transplants, 116, 119–122
Treadmills, 85
Triglycerides, 5–6, 19, 21t, 25
Type I diabetes; See Insulin-
  dependent diabetes
Type II diabetes; See Non-insulin-
  dependent diabetes

U Underwater weighing, 27

V Vascular disease, peripheral, 118–119
VCRs, 87–88
Vision loss, retinopathy and, 117
VO$_2$ max
  and aerobic capacity, 22–23, 66
  exertion levels and, 35–39

W Walking, 40t, 66–67, 122
  interval walking, 118–119
  for senior citizens, 107
Warm-ups, 61
Water, fluid replacement and, 132–133
Water exercises, 40t, 70, 110, 115,
  117, 118
Water sports, high-risk, 137–138
Water walking, 70, 110, 115
Weather conditions, exercise safety
  and, 64, 107

Weight control/reduction, 2, 6,
  91–103
  for beginners, 93–97
  body fat composition, 15–16, 25–30
  diabetes/body weight link, 92–93
  and diet changes, 99–103
  dieting myths, 97–98
  hunger and exercise, 97
  intensive insulin therapy and, 93
Weight lifting; see Strength training
Work, rate of, 39; See also METs

Y Yoga, 83